D1232355

STOP YOUR BITCHING
THE STEP BY STEP GUIDE TO BALANCE HORMONES AND END PMS & MENSTRUAL CRAMPS

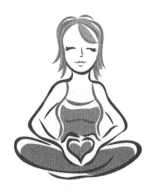

By
Cathy Margolin, L.Ac. Dipl. OM
Copyright 2013

ISBN 978-0-9899467-1-1

Printed in the United State of America

Margolin, Cathy
Stop Your Bitching   A Step By Step Guide to Balance Hormones & End PMS & Menstrual Cramps
ISBN- 978-0-9899467-1-1
To order, please call 877-818-9990 or visit
Shop.PacHerbs.com
Email inquiries to: info@PacHerbs.com

Cover design, layout and illustrations by Lynda Modaff
@ psychicdogart.com

GET THE GUIDEBOOK

30 DAYS OF TIPS TO:

STOP YOUR BITCHING

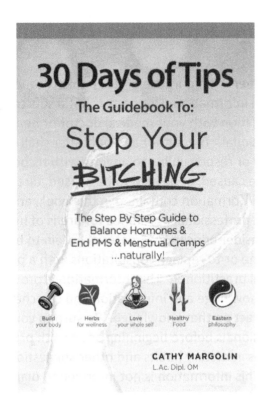

30 Days of Tips

The Guidebook To:

Stop Your
BITCHING

The Step By Step Guide to
Balance Hormones &
End PMS & Menstrual Cramps
...naturally!

| Build your body | Herbs for wellness | Love your whole self | Healthy Food | Eastern philosophy |

CATHY MARGOLIN
L.Ac. Dipl. OM

Cathy Margolin has been committed to Complementary Medicine for over thirty years. While raising two children and coping with her parents health challenges she became frustrated with Western medicine's lack of preventative care. She turned to Alternative and Complementary Medicine therapies such as herbal medicine, acupuncture, healthy foods and nutrition. She is a Licensed Acupuncturist and Herbalist in Los Angeles, California. She completed her undergraduate studies at SMU in Texas, with a BA Degree and BBA Degree. Her Masters Degree is in Oriental Medicine from Emperors College in Santa Monica, California. Cathy has been given the honor of "Distinguished Alumni" from Emperors College and is also recognized as a Diplomat in Oriental Medicine with the National Certification Commission for Acupuncture and Oriental Medicine. Cathy has a private acupuncture and herbal practice in Beverly Hills, California. Cathy is the founder of Pacific Herbs, an herbal wellness company providing the highest quality Traditional Chinese Medicine herbal products.

Acknowledgements

This book started as a passing thought and became this reality after years of discussions and contemplation. I want to thank all those who helped along the way. All the moms and dads I've counseled and women of all ages who have shared their health challenges with me. Thanks to all those who believed this information was worth sharing and to those who made it a physical reality. Thank you to Jennifer, my colleague and Gabby, my editor. You guys rock. My mom was the ultimate inspiration and her eternal lessons I will forever appreciate. My father allowed me to be me and whose memory still inspires me to always make time for contagious laughs. My daughters, whom I will always love and adore. You teach me new lessons everyday. Thank you for your honest feedback and for allowing me to ask your friends to also give their input along the way. The biggest thank you to my husband. Your never ending support and confidence made this and so many other projects a reality. I love you and I couldn't do it without you.

Start Here

**Welcome to YOUR Step By Step Guide
To Balance Your Hormones And End
PMS & Menstrual Cramps.**

There are 10 Chapters.

**Read one chapter each day for the next 10
days and do the "Your Part" at the end of
each chapter in a note book you create.
Nothing fancy just a place to write a few
things down.**

**It's YOUR body and you must complete
each "YOUR PART" at the end of each
chapter to create the healthy body you
want.**

**Commit the next 10 days
to learning how you can change
YOUR health for a lifetime.**

**(Rather than skipping ahead, read this book one
chapter at a time! There is a lot to think about
each day. Each chapter needs a 24 hour
"digestive" time before you move on. If you
move to quickly you may miss the full benefits of
"YOUR PART". Give yourself time.)**

Table of Contents

"You have brains in your head.
You have feet in your shoes.
You can steer yourself any
direction you choose."
Dr. Seuss

Own Up

If your life is often at the mercy of your monthly menstrual cycle, then this is your guide to pain-free "Periods". If your life is ruled by "The Pill" (that you would prefer not to take), this is your guide to freedom from "The Pill".

My inspiration to write this book came after suffering from debilitating menstrual pain as a teenager. After seeing my own daughters have the same type of pain, and hearing stories from my patients who were suffer with monthly menstrual pain, I decided to create a fun way to learn how to end the cycle of suffering. Missing school, work or any activity each month because of your menstrual cycle does not have to be your "normal" routine.

This book will give you the knowledge and power to change this cycle of pain.

Throughout this book you will be introduced to natural alternatives for menstrual cramps and PMS (pre-menstrual syndrome.) Because Western medical schools do not teach 90% of what is introduced in this book, you will likely encounter unfamiliar jargon as you read. This is also why you will not hear these alternatives from your Western doctor.

Don't worry, it will all be explained in non-medical terms and you will have a newly found education about your body and a new found empowerment from this education.

One of my first patients was Lisa. Lisa was a 15 year old young woman. Each month for the past 3 years she would miss school at the start of her period. Her cramps were so intense she started popping NSAID's (pain killers) at the first hint of pain. Sometimes the pain was so intense she would vomit. Usually she had no appetite and didn't eat. Either way her stomach was in knots. She couldn't study so she was always getting behind in her school work. The only thing that helped a little was a heating pad, lots of pain killers and staying in bed. It was the same story every month.
Lisa knew I was studying Chinese Medicine and asked if there was anything that could help. I treated her with Acupuncture, herbs and lifestyle changes eight years ago. She has not needed to use oral contraception or NSAID's pain killers and has normal, pain free menstrual cycles ever month.

If you follow the guidelines in this book you too can "normalize" your hormonal cycles and have pain free periods. When your hormones are balanced your body functions smoothly, you have lots of energy, a strong immune and digestive system, you sleep well and you have a strong sex drive.

Let's get started on this journey together. I'm excited you have decided to explore the options and Stop Your Bitching... naturally!

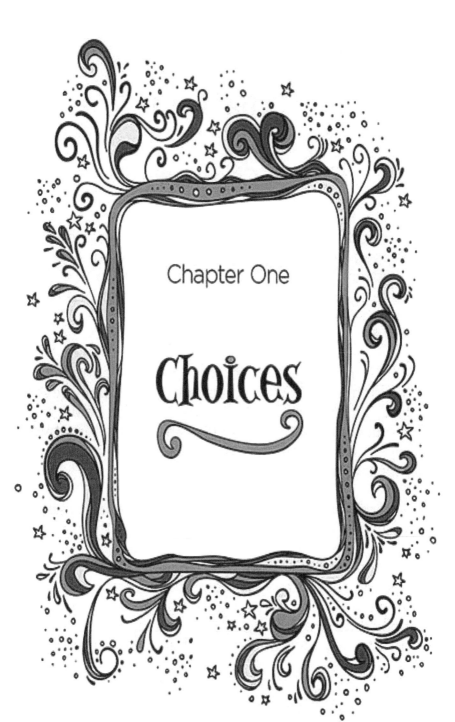

Chapter One

Choices

Chapter 1

Choices

Our bodies' natural hormonal rhythm should happen naturally, with us barely noticing, like breathing. Some women seem lucky, they don't have period pain and barely notice their monthly periods, while others try everything yet continue to suffer.

This handbook is written for those suffering and seeking a natural alternative to period pain beyond birth control pills and over-the-counter pain medications, which are often the only alternatives for primary dysmenorrhea otherwise known as monthly period cramps.

The rhythms of your hormones can compromise your overall health. A dysfunctional pattern can often be a result of a combination of factors. Adolescence brings many changes to a girl's body, but the root of the problems may have started while you were in the womb and growing up. Your body's natural hormonal balance can be severely affected by food and many chemicals you were exposed to that you may not even know about! Don't bother trying to place blame or point fingers, let's move on to fixing the problem. You are making a choice to change! You can fix, re-create and revamp the rest of your life starting now. What happened yesterday is in the past. Today is a new day.

If your period pain is unbearable and you succumb to taking Non-Steroidal Anti-Inflammatory Drugs, otherwise known as NSAID's such as Tylenol, Advil, Motrin or the generic ibuprofen and acetaminophen products to get through a day of bleeding, I want you to know... you do have other choices! Temporary painkillers like NSAID's which are harmful to both your liver, kidneys and your GI (gastrointestinal tract, depending on which over-the-counter brand your taking).

There are other choices that will treat the root of your pain and help you feel normal again. The choices you make when you are young, particularly under the age of 18, are **especially important** because you are still in a small window of important development years. Health at this age is critical to vibrant health later in life.

You have chosen to do something different. Here's your guide to CHANGE!

Change the way you feel each month when your menstrual cycle arrives. Change daily habits to improve your health all month long.
Change is the one constant in a girl's body, understanding THAT makes everything else easy.

Healing starts from within so you must begin with an attitude change. This will play a huge role in your healing. Take charge; It's up to you and only you. Your bodies dis-ease (lack of comfort) is not completely dependent upon your genes or your DNA. Don't ever believe you are completely tied to your genetics. The idea that just because your mother, grandmother or sisters have terrible debilitating monthly period pain doesn't mean you will too. The mentality that your curse is part of your DNA, is wrong. Don't allow your DNA to define your future.

You are going to have to make life style changes, but it will always be your choice. If you want a quick fix to mask your menstrual symptoms then a pill may be the right choice for you. If you want to do what's natural and healthy for your body, then you must accept that making life style choices are an integral part of the plan. Just give yourself a little time, one step at a time, and you will see lasting health.

Your Part 1

Visualize yourself having pain free periods. What would you do on that day? See yourself doing these things.
You will make this happen!

Start each day or end each day with a 1-minute visualization with 2 extra days each month that you now own.

Pretend every month is now 33 days long...
Not the usual 30 or 31...

Write down what you will do with this extra time. For example..."Sunday, I visualize myself doing...?" See yourself doing this either before going to sleep each night or before getting out of bed each morning.

Visualize every day for at least a month. Make it a new ritual. Rituals will become important parts of your life. You may eventually skip the writing down part...but you must still perform the visualization.

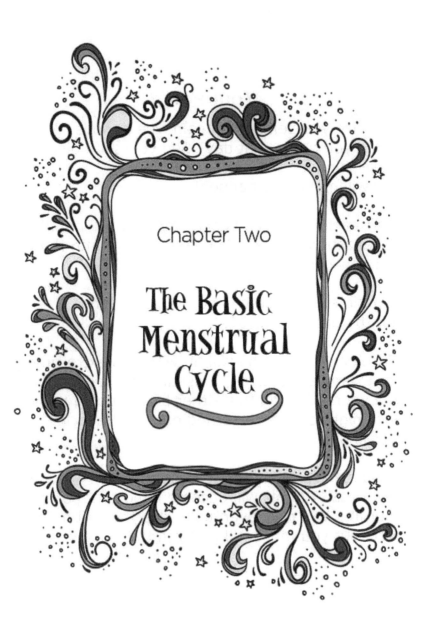

Chapter Two

The Basic Menstrual Cycle

Chapter 2

The Basic Menstrual Cycle

Let's start with a basic understanding of your monthly cycle. Some of you may want to skip this section, totally understandable; chances are you've heard it before. But don't, because I refer back to this later in the book. If you stay with me here you'll find I keep it fairly basic. Even modern medicine has a hard time understanding why we menstruate. Did you know we are the only mammals that have a "monthly" cycle?

Understanding the menstrual cycle gives you insight into your body's natural rhythms. With this knowledge comes empowerment.

Here's a brief overview of a woman's menstrual cycle. The goal here is to give you enough details to empower you while at the same time keeping it simple.

A 28 day menstrual cycle on a graph is shown below. I am trying to keep it fairly simplified. If you want more information the internet has literally thousands of websites that will explain your menstrual cycle in more detail.

Hormones are amazing chemicals that are basically the body's messengers. Hormones are made up of proteins or steroids and are secreted directly into our bloodstream. They keep our body functioning correctly and we couldn't survive without them (some of us think we can barely survive with them!). Some of their major roles include regulating metabolism, reproduction and responses to stress. Our hormonal cycles can make us an emotional mess. Is this just part of being born with ovaries and a uterus?- I don't believe it has to be. You can take back control and keep control of your hormones once you understand the process. I call this, "keeping your hormones on a short lease and house trained."

Learn the steps here and you will have control of your monthly hormonal cycles.

Even though its your hypothalamus and pituitary glands (both in the brain) that are sending the hormonal signals back and forth to your ovaries and you're not consciously aware of this, it doesn't mean these signals have to be totally out of your control. Yes your body wants to constantly prepare for pregnancy. Without this programming our species would be infertile and none of us would be here. Your body is doing what nature intends it to do: procreate, prepare for babies and make babies.

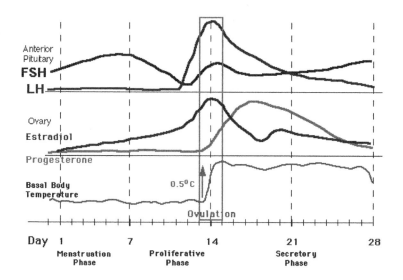

Day 1   7   14   21   28

Menstruation Phase   Proliferative Phase   Secretory Phase

Now lets see what a typically, woman's monthly hormone fluctations look like and what it means to us everyday.

Personally I never really liked the chart! In fact the lines all over the place totally confuse me for all most of my life. So I created an easier way to understand what your body is doing each month. I've written it as a play with a cast of characters.

HERE IS THE "PLAY"
"YOUR MONTHLY "CYCLE"

Imagine it's a play and two hormones, Estrogen and Progesterone, play the leading roles in this reproduction cycle. We'll call them Ester and Terone. The three supporting cast members are also hormones, but act more like messengers, Leu, Francis and Mr. T.

Meet the Cast of Hormone Characters:

Ester -The Leading Lady = Estrogen
(Estrogen is really made up of three chemicals Estrone, Estradiol and Estriol, but let's keep it simple and just call her Ester.) Ester always wants to have a baby and works hard all month long to prepare for a new life to grow inside her.

Terone - The Happy Leading Man = Progesterone
Terone is a happy go lucky kind of guy. But he's a bit confusing. He's both a manly man yet his feelings can get hurt easily and will quietly drop out of the picture if he doesn't feel needed (ie: if there's no baby, he's not needed).

Leu - The Messenger = Luteinizing Hormone
This story has a messenger named Leu whose main job is telling us when to release an egg from our ovaries each month.

Francis - The Brainiac = FSH hormone or Follicle Stimulating Hormone.
A follicle is what we call our eggs before they are fully mature. Francis comes from the pituitary gland which is located in our brains; she also acts as a messenger.

Mr. T – Small But Important Part = Testosterone

Yes, women have this hormone too. Mr. T makes us feel beautiful and sexy. He gives us muscle mass and makes our day when he arrives. We don't have much testosterone but what we have gives us a zest for life.

Sperm= Male sperm
Egg = Female egg

So those are the main players and like any good play, things can get complicated. These players interact in different ways. Sometimes when one is not feeling quite right or doesn't "show" to the party, it throws the rest of the cast out of balance.

For example

When Francis (our brainiac) studies too much, she gets completely stressed out and can't play her role. If Leu decides not to come to opening night, it's hard for the show to go on. If Terone is too weak to support his leading lady, things don't flow so well. If Ester becomes too domineering and decides to boss Terone around, again imbalance, disharmony and nobody gets along.

Ester our leading lady (estrogen) is the key player. She is dominant for the first 14 days of the monthly cycle, but after approximately day 17 she needs to drop out of sight and allows Terone to dominate and be the leading hormone until your period starts once again. If Terone cannot or does not play this role, other problems will develop. If Ester stays on stage and dominates Terone, everything is thrown off and problems begin.

As I mentioned, a woman's body is always preparing for pregnancy. Our bodies remind me of the Girl Scout motto, "Be Prepared". That's what we naturally do each month. We prepare for pregnancy whether fertilization is going to happen or not.

Here's the basic "Play" your body performs each month.

THE PLAY "YOUR CYCLE" BEGINS

Prologue: Bleeding starts on day one of the month. You are not up for partying, let alone school or work, so you struggle through your day and bleed. All the cast members, including our leading lady Ester, just stay home (Blood levels of estrogen are lowest on the first day of your period).

Scene One:

It is day 3 and you are beginning to feel a bit more like yourself again. Ester wants to go out and play now that the overall "crummy" feeling has subsided. Ester begins to build up in our blood.

Scene Two:

It is day 6 (approximately) of the month and now that the bleeding has ended Francis, our brainiac, instinctively knows that it is time to make way for a baby. She tells Ester to start making plans for a baby. Ester starts hitting the gym to build up, she goes everyday for 2 weeks. She knows the follicle (immature egg) will soon arrive from the ovaries and she needs to prepare the womb.

Scene Three:

It is day 13 of our month long play and Ester has increased in strength (check the chart, she's nearly at an all-time high). Now the time has come for Leu's big moment on stage. He has a very important message. He tells the ovaries about Ester building up and feeling good. Leu says now is the best time to release an egg from one of the ovaries. Ester wants a baby to be implanted in her uterus. Side note: When Ester is peaking, you feel good and look good, most likely because estrogen is also known to affect skin tone. But this estrogen peak may also cause some confusion: cravings for sweet or salty foods, restlessness, even anxious feelings. This high level of estrogen is usually only sustained for a 24-48 hour period.

Scene Four:

It is Day 13, Terone (also known as Mr. Happy) comes on stage. When Terone is strong, we often feel stronger and more beautiful. He's been watching from back stage and patiently waiting for something to do. Now is his moment and he wants to strut his stuff. When the mature follicle (now called an egg) was released from the ovary Terone got his queue to also hit the gym and build up. He knows pregnancy depends on him being strong. He only has a short window of time (a couple of days) till he hits his peak. Mr. T also makes a brief appearance here. His presence helps us feel strong. We have more of a "zest" for life when he is present.

SCENE FIVE:

It is Day 18, the sun is shining today and Terone is going out to play. Terone makes us feel good, though we may be a bit bossy and push others around. Terone tells the uterus to fill with blood and prepare for pregnancy. Ester likes this because she's always hoping for a baby, wondering if this will be the month. While Terone is peaking we normally feel a greater sense of well being, even euphoria.

SCENE SIX:

It is Day 25 and Ester is irritable. She's snapping at everyone because she has the worst headache. On top of that, she is complaining that she gained weight, despite all the exercise she's been doing and her breasts are getting sore. She is thinking she could be pregnant but she's not really sure.

Scene Seven:

Now it's Day 27 and alas sperm's timing was off, and he didn't meet egg. Everyone is a little disappointed, pregnancy didn't happen this month. Ester has stopped going to the gym, she's weaker now. Terone quietly leaves the stage realizing nobody needs him. Now all that blood in the lining of the uterus is not needed. It begins dying and prepares to leave, naturally. You are feeling a little glum because Terone is gone. The imbalance or sudden decrease of Terone makes you a little more fragile. A good cry might feel good just about now. Terone decreasing suddenly seems to cause a distortion of reality triggering all kinds of emotions: depression, anxiety, hurt, confusion, frustration and irritability. This is the worst possible day to get a parking ticket or hear anything you might construe as negative about you.

Finale:

Day 28 your period begins again and you begin to bleed. Of course you know I've simplified the process, and there is more to hormone production than I've mentioned above. Our adrenal glands, (small walnut-sized hormone factories) which sit on top of our kidneys are involved. These glands produce a chemical called cortisol which regulates female hormones, especially progesterone (Terone). Our adrenals can be affected by our thyroid gland in our neck and lots of other thins so you can see the picture is more complex than just throwing a few switches to turn things on and off. When one player is absent, a whole chain of events may not happen the way it should.

One other note, not everyone has a "perfect" 28 day menstrual cycle. Normal can mean 25 to 35 day cycles, so don't stress over your cycle being exact each month. Actors can't always be on time, it's just the nature of the business. The endocrine system in the body is complicated. It includes the hypothalamus, thyroid, pituitary, ovaries, parathyroid, pancreas and adrenal cortex and medulla, all which produce hormones in women. Stress can interfere with all of these functions. Stressors include emotional stress, dietary stress and inflammatory stress. I will address these aspects in later chapters.

This cycle, "This Play" is like a You Tube video played thousands of times. It's pretty much the same thing, but varies with outside influences that change as our lives change. Stress, weight, sleep, exercise, food (particularly junk food), drugs, chemicals in our foods and products we use, alcohol consumption and birth control pills all make it difficult for our players, our main actors Ester, Terone, Leu and Francis to carry on their roles like they should.

As I previously mentioned, we women are all about change. We are always in a cycle of change and this is natural. Your cycle will often change with age and before and after child birth. Nothing ever stays completely the same when it comes to a womens body.

Women who experience low progesterone (our character Terone, in relation to estrogen, Ester) or fluctuating progesterone levels tend to bleed heavily and have irregular cycles. This is common for teenagers as well as women in their 40's as they approach menopause. An over abundance of estrogen in relation to progesterone causes a host of problems; this is discussed in the next chapter.

Your Part 2

The cycle of change happens whether you know about it or not. You didn't decide how and when your menstrual cycle would first arrive; your body decided and then told you by bleeding. Now it's up to you to understand this mystery guest and take control of it before it takes control of you.

Become familiar with the players in the monthly "Play" and do more reading about them so you feel comfortable with the changes your body goes through each month. If you don't yet completely understand your monthly cycle, read more about it on the internet or any number of great women's health books.

Don't skip this step as it will help you have a better overall understanding of your body and how the things you do everyday have long term effects.Buy a wall calendar, one with big boxes that you can write on and make notes.

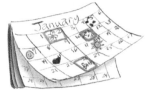 I like this method over a date book or diary because it's easy to refer back to it and it will give you an accurate picture over time. You can easily flip through the months, a year from now, and see what your cycle

was like. Trying to remember all these little details is impossible. But a calendar takes seconds to fill in and will provide a wealth of knowledge down the road.

Mark the calendar in red for the days you're bleeding and everything else in other colors. You will also start tracking your emotional symptoms. When you feel emotionally unstable, depressed, happy or extremely energetic and positive, write it down. You can create a little system of smiley faces or stars or whatever works for you. Be as creative or uncreative as you desire. No one else needs to see the calendar.

Is your monthly cycle regular or irregular? Bleeding every 28 days is considered the norm, but few people experience this month after month. As you track your cycle on the wall calendar for the next few months count the number of days between bleeding and mark this at the top of each month.

As you read the next few chapters you will begin to understand how hormone fluctuations are affecting your moods and you will be able to see how your cycle plays a part. This calendar will become your new BFF. Another option is to use an App on your phone. These can be fairly easy and convenient. Either option will work, as long you keep it up to date.

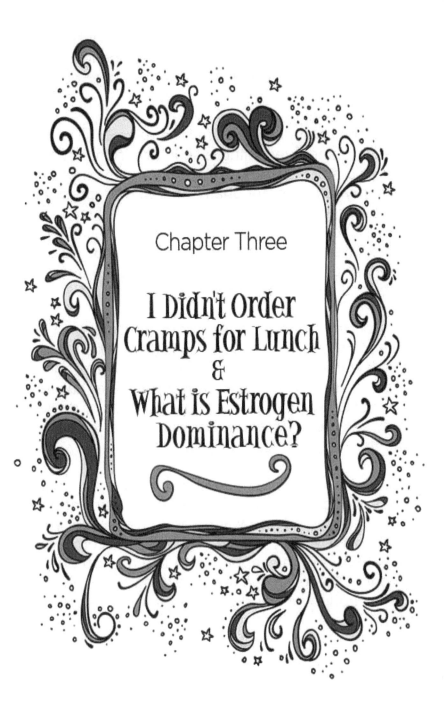

Chapter Three

I Didn't Order
Cramps for Lunch
&
What is Estrogen
Dominance?

Chapter 3

I Didn't Order Cramps for Lunch
&
What is Estrogen Dominance?

Cramps are a symptom of something not working correctly in your body. This pain is simply our body's way of crying out for help.

Mainstream medicine often treats pain symptoms by hiding them with pain killers, thus suppressing symptoms rather than looking for the root cause.

What if we approach pain from a different perspective? What if we look at pain as a gift rather than a curse? Pain is our body telling us something isn't working quite right and we need an adjustment. When we listen to little pains we often can avoid the bigger ones that inevitably follow.

If you're a soccer player and you sprain your ankle but continue to play soccer, your ankle pain will increase. Your little sprain will become more inflamed and more troublesome because you missed the message your body was sending. Let's say you decide to run a marathon on your sprained ankle, how will it feel upon finishing? You get the picture.

You can block messages on your phone, in your email and in your body, but doing so does not mean the messages were not sent. You cannot cure the underlying imbalance by blocking out pain messages.

A primary cause of painful menstrual cramps is prostaglandins. I promised only a small amount of necessary medical terminology, hang in there, it's not to complicated an explaination. These naturally occurring fatty acids are higher in some women. They cause cramps and may also be the cause of heavy menstrual bleeding.

Prostaglandins are chemicals released from cells of the uterus as we bleed, or discard the uterine lining (our periods). Prostaglandins are not hormones, but they act like messengers similar to the way hormones do. They differ from hormones because they are produced in various places throughout the body, and they target cells in their immediate vicinity with a very specific function. In the uterus, prostaglandins causes both unterine inflammation and the contraction and constriction of blood flow to the uterine, in other words,

Cramps!   This in turn causes the lining of the uterus to break down and die and this is our PERIOD
.
These contractions, of the uterus, in many ways are our bodies practicing labor contractions so the uterus will be strong and ready for childbirth. Your body is smarter than you might think.

However, even though modern medicine can pinpoint these prostaglandin chemicals as the cause of cramps, suppressing them as we so often do with NSAID's is only a band-aid to the underlying problem. As you will soon discover, hormonal imbalance is the real root of the problem not just prostaglandins. Sheilding us from the prostaglandin message with NSAID's creates a host of other problems as you will see in the next chapter.

A Little More Details On Cramps

Period pain, or uterine cramps, is categorized by Western medicine as primary dysmenorrhea (PD) and characterized by severe uterine pain during menstruation. While most women experience minor pain during menstruation. PD is diagnosed when the pain is so severe as to limit normal activities, or require medication. Pain may precede menstruation by several days or may accompany it, and it usually subsides as menstruation tapers off.

Secondary dysmenorrhea is diagnosed when symptoms are attributable to an underlying disease, disorder, or structural abnormality either within or outside the uterus. When secondary dysmenorrhea is the cause of menstrual cramps you should consult with a MD, General Practitioner, or Gynecologist for your best treatment options. I would also recommend consulting with a registered nurse or nurse practitioner because they will often spend much more time with you and are more knowledgeable about complementary therapies including diet and supplements.

What is Estrogen Dominance and is it causing my painful cramps?

The term "estrogen dominance" was coined by the late Dr. John Lee. He describes this condition as having deficient, normal or excessive estrogen in relation to progesterone. This means even if you have just a small amount of estrogen throughout your monthly cycle, but you have little to no progesterone, you can still be estrogen dominant. Keep in mind, it is the balance of these two hormones that matters more than the actual amount. As you saw in "The Play", the amounts fluctuate all month long, so measuring these amounts can get very tricky.

Many chemicals in our environment behave as estrogens. You may also hear this referred to as "unopposed estrogen". We are exposed to these chemicals all our lives, including in the womb. (Remember I mentioned in the 1st Chapter your hormone levels may be in flux at birth and even before you entered puberty.) This group of chemicals has been given the name "Xenoestrogens" (Xeno is the Greek word for stranger).

These "stranger" chemicals accumulate in our bodies as we develop and age. To our bodies, Xenoestrogens look like estrogen and both men and women are at risk.

Our fat cells can store these xeno-estrogen mimicking chemicals. Storehouses of these xeno's can reduce our excretion of copper. (copper is a trace mineral, or one which we have a very small amount of in our bodies). If we don't excrete enough copper we can create a copper accumulation or excess.

Why is this important? Copper accumulation disables certain vitamins and minerals, namely iron, zinc, vitamin C and E. You'll see why these are important in the chapter on supplements.

Remember in the "PLAY" our two leading cast members Ester and Terone need to stay in balance and work together for everything in our body to work optimally. If Ester is dominant and does not give Terone some of the spotlight for at least 10-

14 days of our monthly cycles, then things don't play out the way they should. Ester should not play a dominant role all month long. You will see in later chapters how diet, exercise and supplements and even changing your laundry detergent can reduce estrogen dominance, and thereby reduce your menstrual cramps and other PMS symptoms.

If you are experiencing any of these symptoms, then it is likely that Ester (Estrogen) dominates your monthly hormonal cycle.

Here's An A-Z List of Estrogen Dominate Symptoms

Acceleration of aging, menstruation begins at younger age
Agitation or Anxiety
Allergy (asthma, hives, rashes, sinus congestion)
Autoimmune disorders Lupus, Thyroiditis (Hashimoto's)
Breast cancer (men and women)
Breast tenderness with period
Cervical dysplasia (abnormal papsmear)
Cold hands and feet
Copper excess
Decreased sex drive
Depression with anxiety or agitation
Dry eyes
Endometriosis
Fat gain around abdomen hips and thighs
Fatigue

Fibrocystic (lumpy breasts)
Fibroids
Foggy thinking
Gall bladder disease
Hair loss
Headaches
Hypoglycemia (low blood sugar)
Increased blood clotting
Infertility
Irregular menstrual periods
Irritability
Insomnia
Magnesium deficiency
Memory loss
Mood swings
Osteoporosis
Ovarian cancer
Ovarian cysts
PMS/PMT
Polycystic ovaries
Pre-menopausal bone loss
Prostrate cancer (in men)
Sluggish metabolism
Thyroid dysfunction
Uterine cancer
Water retention, bloating and Zinc deficiency

Western medicine tests are available to test estrogen and other hormone levels. This might be done by testing your blood, saliva and/or urine.

As an Oriental medicine doctor I generally do not look at the outcome of lab tests, but rather I diagnosis according to patterns, including those patterns and symptoms that look like estrogen dominance. If an excess of symptoms are present, then the imbalance is present. It is as simple and straightforward as that. If your health professional believes you absolutely need a blood, saliva or urine test to check your estrogen, progesterone and or testosterone levels then that is a decision you need to make with your health professional.

However, you should know that blood tests often times do not give a true picture of how much estrogen is bioavailable (at the tissue level) in your body. A blood test is a snap shot in time and a woman's estrogen level changes every six to eighteen hours, as does her progesterone levels. You read about daily changes in Chapter 2. Not to complicate the issue but, a woman's body also makes approximately 30 different estrogens including the 3 most important ones estrone, estradiol and estriol. The only estrogen tested by a blood test is <u>estradiol</u>.

I am trained to read blood tests and when my patients come to me with blood, urine or saliva tests results, I first ask them a plethora of questions about how and when the test was performed. What lab was used? What day of your cycle was the test conducted? Were any drugs taken within the last 5-7 days? Was a base line test done previously? As you see, there are more to test results than just a number on a piece of paper. More often than not, my patient did not track her cycle, but rather went for the test on the first available appointment. Your health provider may recommend a saliva test on day 21 of your cycle (when progesterone should be peaking), 24-hour urine tests on day 3 of your cycle (my recommendation), or look only at blood tests.

Try this online quiz and find out if your hormones are in balance or out of balance.
www.womeninbalance.org/pdf/quiz.pdf

One last comment on estrogen. Estrogen dominance is more than a list of possible symptoms. It can wreak real havoc every day of our lives. Cells grow more rapidly when estrogen, rather than progesterone, is present. Progesterone is a hormone that keeps cells orderly. It stops growth, induces cell maturity and programmed cell death. Normal levels of progesterone are nature's protectors. We know natural progesterone levels can actually protect us from some cancers.

Consider that we know estrogen stimulates cell division and growth in the breasts. This is the very reason many therapies for breast cancer are targeted towards stopping estrogen production. For some breast cancer patients this means a hysterectomy, including the removal of the ovaries, even before menopause. Drugs called LH (luteinizing hormone) inhibitors are also commonly used to stop the production of estrogen in breast cancer treatments. Additionally, drugs such as Tamoxifen, which block estrogen receptors, are another method to lower estrogen levels.

My Patient Linda:

Linda was 20 when she came to me for help with her horrible back pain and period cramps. She always had debilitating cramps from the onset of her period. During her teen years she dosed herself with over the counter pain killers. During college she tried the birth control pill because all of her friends told her it was the answer to her painful periods. By her third month on the pill Linda found herself more depressed than ever in her life. She was more moody and couldn't seem to control her feelings, even crying often which was unusual for her. She was unhappy with the 5-10 pounds she gained quickly and just didn't quite feel "right." But her periods were lighter and more pain free than ever so she decided to continue the birth control pills.

When she came home for the summer her mother noticed her depression worsening. Linda went off the pill and started to exercise and watch her diet. She came to me for acupuncture and herbs and we discussed her other options. Linda decided to supplement her diet and make the changes I suggested while stopping the birth control pill. Within two months of being off the pill she had dropped the weight she had gained and felt more at ease. The moodiness and depression were getting better and the acupuncture and life style changes were making a difference in her monthly cramps.

Today, Linda is 25 and says she would never again use the pill. The depression she experienced when taking the pill was unprecedented in her life and even though her doctor had prescribed a low dose pill she really noticed the effects once she stopped taking it. Linda is one example of young women I've worked with who looked for options to alleviate painful periods and after trying the pill, began an alternative path to healing from within.

Your Part 3

Recognize pain is your friend. Be grateful for these early warning signals that your body sends you. Your body is an intelligent machine perfected throughout millions of years of survival in the wild. Trust your body is giving intelligent signals and start listening to them.

Write down each time you listened to your body.

DATE:_____Describe Pain or discomfort

_____

DATE:_____Describe Pain or discomfort

_____

DATE:_____Describe Pain or discomfort

_____

Make your own list and give yourself lots of space.

You will soon make this a healthy habit. Keep track of the number of symptoms from the Estrogen Dominance list that you get each month. If you have more than 3 symptoms each month, consider finding ways to reduce your estrogen dominance. This is explained in later chapters (especially Chapter 6) in more detail.

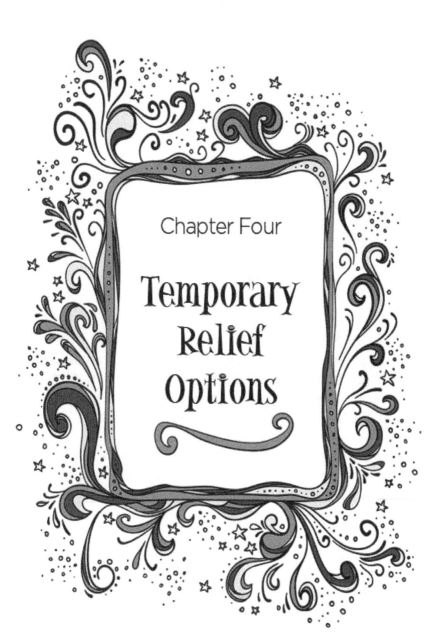

Chapter Four

Temporary Relief Options

Chapter 4

Temporary Relief Options

What are your options to minimize or end painful periods?

Your options can be listed on one hand (almost). But each one is more complex than initially meets the eye. We will explore each in depth in the next few chapters over the next few days.

Here are the options available:

1. Do nothing!
2. Take NSAIDS.
   (Non-Steroidal Anti-Inflammatory Drugs) Discussed here.
3. Take oral contraception. (discussed in Chap. 5)
4. Make lifestyle changes. (see Chapter. 6)
5. Take herbs and vitamins supplements
   (see Chapter. 7 & 8)
6. See alternative practitioners: Acupuncturists, Chiropractors, Homeopathic & Naturopathic doctors. (see Chapter 9)
7. Combine any or all of the above. (Chapter 10)

OPTION #1

#1 Do nothing, is not really an option and you wouldn't be reading this if that was your choice.

Thank goodness you have moved past this option and are ready for real solutions. Give yourself a pat on the back and a lot of credit for deciding to take action and change your life. You deserve it!

Option #2

<u>Taking NSAID's</u> Non-steroidal Anti-Inflammatory Drug's such as ibuprofen (Advil®, Motrin®, Midol PMS®), naproxen (Aleve®), and acetaminophen (Tylenol®) and aspirin. NSAID's are available over the counter with the above names or they are sold under other generic brand names. All have analgesic effects, (pain killers), antipyretic effects, (fever reducing) and in high enough doses anti-inflammatory effects, otherwise known as reducing inflammation.

HOW DO NSAID'S WORK?
WHY ARE THEY SO POPULAR?

Acetaminophen blocks production and release of chemicals that cause pain, such as prostaglandins.

We have all probably experienced the effects of NSAID's for ourselves. Whether taken for muscle aches, period pain or headaches NSAID's work quickly and are effective, but at what cost? All NSAID's have side effects and study after study cites everything from peptic ulcers, diarrhea, nausea, liver damage and increased risk of heart disease. Beyond the documented harm that can occur with short term duration of taking NSAID's there is strong evidence that long term harmful effects compound over time with increased dosage and years of use.

NSAID's are metabolized or broken down in our liver and then excreted. Metabolism may differ depending on the individual and accumulation may occur even with normal dosage. Since NSAID's account for approximately 300 million in sales each year in just the U.S., the wide spread use of these drugs has shed light on the adverse drug reactions or ADR's. Stomach upset, gastrointestinal (GI) effects and renal (kidney) effects, liver toxicity and vascular effects, (heart attacks) are the most prevalent adverse reactions.

The potential for acetaminophen to harm the liver is increased when it is combined with alcohol or drugs that also harm the liver. University of California Los Angeles experts warned in January 2010 that combining many pharmaceutical drugs such as Vicodin and Percocet for pain with an OTC cold and flu medicine can be a deadly liver cocktail. New data is surfacing as liver transplants hit an all time high in the U.S. It turns out the number one cause of liver damage is acetaminophen poisoning from long term overdosing. Unfortunately, most people never knew they were taking too much.

I'm certain many people don't mean to overdose, but did you realize only two extra strength tablets or 650 milligrams daily is the USA. FDA recommended dose? This lower and safer dosage (down from 1000 mg) was recommended by the FDA's own advisory board in June 2009 but has not been completely put into effect by the FDA as of this book printing.

Are you using an acetaminophen sleep aid and an extra strength pain reliever for menstrual cramps? You may be causing liver damage. This information has not been widely publicized. You can check out the Food & Drug Administration website for more information. In addition, new information from the FDA has been released confirming there is no sleep benefit from night time sleep aid products containing acetaminophen and diphenhydramine combinations. Not all drugs are marked, so check with your pharmacist.

You should be aware that combining acetaminophen products may put you over the "safe" dosage recommendations. For example, if you combine any OTC sinus caplet, cold and flu formula, a pain reliever, Sudafed®, Excedrin®, Tylenol®, Pamprin®, Benadryl®, Premsyn®, CVS® decongestant, Eckerd® Pain relief, Thera flu ®cold packets, Vicks® Dayquil or Nyquil, or arthritis pain relief caplets , you're most likely going over the recommended/safe zone for acetaminophen. You guessed it: liver damage.

It may be difficult to consider liver damage as a side effect of one of the most popular drugs OTC (Tylenol) for pain, but it is also the number one cause of liver transplantation surgeries in the U.S. and Europe.

Consider this disturbing quote: "Unfortunately, the prevalence of acetaminophen makes it easy to accidentally exceed the recommended levels, which can occur by dosing more frequently than indicated or by combining two or more acetaminophen-containing products. "   The maximum adult dose is 3 grams per day; toxic daily levels range from 7 to 10 grams per day.

More at this reference:
http://livertox.nlm.nih.gov/Acetaminophen.htm

Ibuprofen based NSAID's

Stomach upset or indigestion is the common side-effect with Ibuprofen based NSAID's. Hundreds of thousands of hospitalizations each year result from overuse of these drugs, many from unnecessary prescriptions. The most common GI problems include, nausea, vomiting, heart burn, bleeding stomach ulcers and diarrhea. Ibuprofen is now required to have the strongest warning given by the FDA on all their products. It's called a "Black Box" warning and looks like this:

Black Box warning on ibuprofen products

Cardiovascular Risk
may incr. risk of serious and potentially fatal cardiovascular thrombotic events, MI, and stroke; risk may incr. w/ duration of use; possible incr. risk if cardiovascular dz or cardiovascular dz risk factors; contraindicated for CABG peri-operative pain

GI Risk
incr. risk serious GI adverse events incl. bleeding, ulcer, and stomach or intestine perforation, which can be fatal; may occur at any time during use and w/o warning sx; elderly pts at greater risk for serious GI events

GI Risks

GI bleeding, ulceration, and stomach or intestinal perforation, which can be fatal may occur at any time and without warning.

Because NSAID's work well at reducing inflammation in the body, by inhibiting prostaglandins, they also inhibit prostaglandins which are beneficial in our GI tracts. This causes an increase in gastric acid, the stomach acid that rises to our esophagus which we know so well as heart burn or GERD (Gastro-Esophageal Reflux Disease).

This has been such a common side effect of NSAID's in fact, that many manufacturers have now created new pills with an "enteric-coating" to minimize stomach upset (GI symptoms). These newer pills don't dissolve in the stomach; rather they begin dissolving in the large intestine in an effort to reduce the risk of stomach ulcers. Unfortunately, these newer pills have other side effects in the large intestines. Bloody diarrhea was noted in a study done in Feb 2010 on some of the newer NSAID's. Another recent study showed over 50% of patients taking NSAIDs have sustained damage to their small intestine.

Ibuprofen NSAIDs should not be used by those suffering from Inflammatory Bowel Disease, Crohn's Disease or Ulcerative Colitis due to their tendency to cause gastric bleeding and form ulceration in the gastric lining.

The use of NSAIDs (except for low-dose aspirin) has been associated with a more than 10-fold increase in heart failure. NSAIDs are also estimated to be responsible for up to 20 percent of hospital admissions for congestive heart failure.

I could not possibly list or site all the studies that have been done on NSAID's, but it's easy to look them up at www.pubmed.com, the largest medical database in the world. Many articles or short abstracts are free. Simply type in "NSAID's" on Google or pubmed.com and start reading. You could be there for days. NSAID's are also associated with kidney problems which can result in high blood pressure and water retention. NSAID's can become toxic to the kidneys if taken concurrently with prescription drugs such as an ACE inhibitor and a diuretic - the so-called "triple whammy" effect. These agents have been shown, quite ironically, to actually increase inflammation (the very thing it's used to treat) when combined with exposure to sunlight.

NSAID's should never be used during pregnancy, particularly during the 3rd trimester. Other common adverse reactions to NSAID's include higher than normal liver enzymes, constipation, headaches and even allergies.

The goal here is not to scare you from ever taking an OTC NSAID ever again... but to impress upon you that just because it's OTC doesn't mean it's completely safe. Depending on your own use and dosage, side effects can be minimized and these products can be used safely. However you should be aware that the use of NSAID's to manage severe menstrual pain each month does carry risks.

A good night's sleep is always a great answer to pain and stress. A trip to a spa would surely help, but it's not always possible. Before you pop that NSAID for a headache or joint pain or period pain, ask yourself where the pain started. What or where did it emanate from? Was it emotional, a fight with a friend? Was it physical, an overworked body? Your body often inherently knows these answers. Key into your own intuitive self and you may be able to CHANGE the behaviors that are requiring you to pop the NSAID's in the first place.

One last comment on NSAID's from an Eastern medicine point of view: we want to minimize liver congestion. "Soothing Liver Qi and moving Liver Blood" is a very important concept in Oriental Medicine. Our liver is the main organ that cleanses our blood and metabolizes every drug we put in our body, including NSAID's. Our liver is therefore very important in menstrual blood flow. Limiting your use of NSAID's may be one of the changes you make to improve your health and well being. I will cover the topic of liver health in the chapter on Oriental medicine.

NIH reference for ibuprofen:
http://livertox.nlm.nih.gov/Ibuprofen.htm

NSAID info graphic here:
www.mercola.com/infographics/nsaids.htm

YOUR PART 4

Every time you take a NSAID write it down for the next few months.

Keep a record so you can be sure you are minimizing your risks. If you don't have this handbook with you when you pop that pill, make a note to yourself in your phone or date book or somewhere so you will remember later to write it down. The only way you will really know how many NSAIDs you take is to keep a detailed record.

Include the brand name or generic name and the dosage you take. At the end of each month add it up and compare it to our safety chart below to keep you in a safe zone for these OTC pain killers.

SAFE CHART FOR NSAID's USE

1 Extra Strength Tylenol for "Muscle Aches & Pains" has 650 mg/milligrams or .650 grams (at the time of this printing)

1000 milligrams = 1 gram   Do not exceed 3 grams per day.
(Divide milligrams by 1000 to convert to grams)
 2 pills = 1250 mg or 1.25 grams
3 pills = 1950 mg or 1.95 grams
4 pills = 2600 mg or 2.6 grams

5 pills = 3250 mg or 3.25 grams (toxic)
6 pills = Toxic Zone above 3 grams

Any more than 5 pills at 650 mg and you are above the 3-gram mark, which The American Liver Foundation recommends you not exceed for any prolonged period of time.

Count and write down how many pills you are taking each month. Damage is cumulative; your liver must to process every single pill.
For example...

Month 1 _____Write down how many NSAID'S you used.

Include the Date / Product Name /Dosage / #of pills used daily.   If it's easier, add this information somewhere in your phone.
It is too difficult to remember how many pills you are taking so   **WRITE IT DOWN** each time. Use this page or create your own record somewhere.

Date	Product Name	Dose in mg	#of pills daily

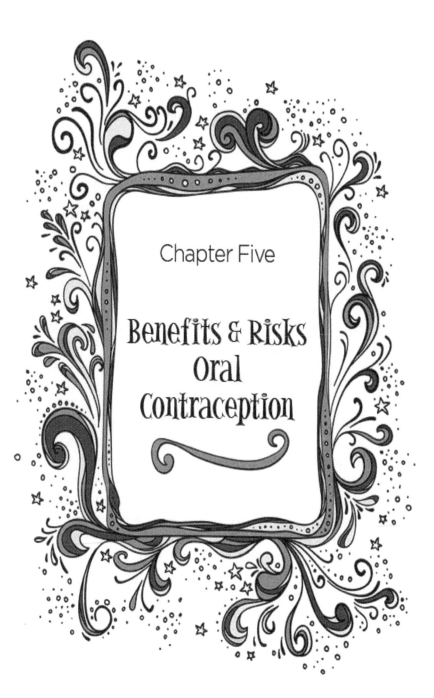

Chapter Five

Benefits & Risks Oral Contraception

Chapter 5

Weigh the Benefits and Risks of The Birth Control Pill

The invention of the birth control pill has given women control over their fertility for the first time in history. Even though indigenous cultures had various means of causing spontaneous abortions, the birth control pill provides freedom from worry over conception unlike anything else.

These little pills have drastically changed women's lives in ways we couldn't have imagined just 50 years ago and in ways we are still discovering. Annual research reveals the benefits and risks of these incredible little pills. Many women choose to use the pill to give them lighter, more manageable, less painful periods. Although there are thousands of studies on the artificial hormones in oral contraception, there is no conclusive evidence that the Pill will repair the underlying mechanisms which are at the root cause of cramps and PMS.

First the facts:

Oral birth control pills or oral contraceptives (OC) are made from synthetic, non-bio-identical hormones with varying degrees of hormone formulations. Some OC's contain both estrogen and progestin while some contain only progestin. Some oral contraceptives have higher or lower doses of these hormones and some may provide doses that change throughout the month. The one common denominator among all oral birth control is the suppression of ovulation. When our bodies are prevented from releasing a follicle that develops into a mature egg each month, fertilization or pregnancy is prevented. OC have an overall effectiveness of 92%- 98% in preventing pregnancy, (depending on who's studies you read). However, statistics on "The Pill's" effect for preventing or relieving menstrual cramps, conducted by the independent Cochrane Collaboration in 2009, which does rigorous reviews, found little evidence that the pill was effective in treating menstrual pain.

The traditional pill mimics your body's 28 day menstrual cycle and contains synthetic hormones for the first 21 days and then placebo pills for seven days. When you're taking the placebo's you have a regular period and bleeding occurs. There are also OC pills available today which prevent all menstrual bleeding. These pills give continuous hormones for a year straight and are called extended cycle birth control. There is also a brand of OC pills on the market that gives you three months of hormones and then a week of placebo or low doses estrogen for planned bleeding during that time. This pill changes your normal menstrual bleeding to four times a year versus the usual thirteen times per year.

"MINI-PILLS"

Also fairly new to the market are what's now referred to as mini-pills. These pills contain only progestin and may be prescribed because a woman is breastfeeding. Estrogen in OC pills has been implicated in reducing breast milk production. Estrogen may also cause nausea when taken. This pill effects the lining of the uterus making it inhospitable for a fertilized egg to implant.

You may want to watch this short video explanation. The Amazing Journey from Egg to Embryo

www.medicinenet.com/conception_pictures_slidesho w/article.htm

Birth control patches and vaginal rings are also made from synthetic hormones and have roughly the same effect as the OC pill. The action of preventing ovulation with synthetic hormones is the same. A slightly higher risk of blood clots has recently been associated with the ring.

Will the Pill help my period cramps?

Many women will tell you their periods are lighter and less painful while taking OC's than before they took the pill. The traditional OC pill has been used to treat medical conditions such as polycystic ovary syndrome (PCOS), endometriosis, adenomyosis, anemia related to menstruation and painful menstruation (dysmenorrhea), dysfunctional uterine bleeding, irregular menstruation and even mild to moderate acne.

Researchers from the Cochrane Library concluded that: "No conclusions can be made about the efficacy of commonly used modern lower dose oral contraceptives for dysmenorrhea (period pain). While there is some evidence from four RCTs that combined oral contraception pills (OCPs) with medium dose of estrogen and 1st/2nd generation progesterone's are more effective than placebo, it should be emphasized that the studies were small, of poor quality and all included much higher doses of hormones that those commonly prescribed today. Therefore no recommendations can be made regarding the efficacy of modern combined oral contraceptives."[12]

The Cochrane Database is an international not-for-profit and independent organization, dedicated to up-to-date, accurate information about the effects of health-care readily available worldwide. The Cochrane Collaboration produces and disseminates systematic reviews of health-care interventions and promotes the search for evidence in the form of clinical trials and other studies of interventions. The *Cochrane Collaboration* was founded in 1993. They publish the Cochrane Database of Systematic Reviews quarterly as part of the Cochrane Library.

It is essential to balance the overall body to balance hormone production levels. Birth control pills do not correct this underlying dysfunction. Birth control pills do inhibit ovulation which reduces the menstrual blood and prostaglandin levels by suppressing endometrial (the uterine lining) tissue growth, however they do Correct the underlying imbalance and dysfunctions will heal.

Do your homework when taking OC or other hormone methods for birth control. Below you will find quotes from some of the largest and most recent scientific studies. Reference links are provided for you to do your own research. I recognize that birth control decisions are personal, and you must choose for yourself. Most doctors do not have time to sit with every patient and explain all the benefits and risks to a given drug, so it's up to you to become an informed consumer. When reading studies on the internet be sure to check who funded the study and if it was "double blind" (In double blind studies neither researchers nor research subjects have the knowledge of who is getting placebo versus real therapies).

Common Side Effects of the Pill

The most common side effects of OC pills include increased vaginal secretions, irregular bleeding, reduced menstrual blood flow, breast tenderness, increase in breast size, decreases in acne, nausea, increases in blood pressure, mood changes, depression, facial skin discoloration, weight gain and headaches and fatal blood clots and break through bleeding (off cycle menstrual bleeding). Oral contraception use has also been associated with increased risks for some cancers, elevated triglycerides and Lupus.

Smoking and the Pill

Oral contraception is particularly dangerous for smokers. Research has shown that smokers over the age of 35 have an increased risk of serious cardiovascular disease when on the pill.

Sexual Dysfunction and the Pill

Testosterone is the hormone which turns on our sex drive. According to a Boston University Medical Center study in 2006, testosterone can be lowered as a result of taking birth control pills and *may stay that way for your entire life*.[13] This is when women are most fertile so it makes perfect sense that nature provides a boost to make us sexually hungry during this time.

Yeast infections and the Pill

"The most common yeast infection is an over growth of a fungus called Candidiasis or thrush. Taking birth control hormones does put you in a higher risk category for susceptibility to Candida infections."[14] The most common symptoms are redness, itching and discomfort. A common cause of vaginal irritation is due to candidiasis also known as vaginitis. A study on 8314 patients concluded "In patients using oral contraceptives (OCs), we found yeast in 28.8% as compared with women of the same age not using OCs (20.3%)."[15]

Digestive Flora and the Pill

Birth control pills are damaging your gut flora. Women who are taking contraceptive pills do profound damage to their internal digestive gut flora. Probiotics can be used to rebuild healthy bacteria and repair gut flora.

Magnesium and Zinc Depletion and the Pill

Magnesium and zinc are essential minerals our bodies need daily. Government research on essential vitamins and minerals has been a hot topic for years to ensure citizens are ingesting foods with the proper amounts. "Overall. . . results indicate that OC use does reduce vitamin nutritional status, protein levels, and levels of some trace minerals." [16] Here is another example: "It was concluded that females consuming OCA (oral contraception agents) should pay particular attention to vitamin and mineral intake and, if warranted, consume physiologic supplements of needed nutrients."[17] There are many more studies with the same conclusions on the US National Library of Medicine, National Institute of Health website at: www.pubmed.com.

Vitamin B Depletion and the Pill

Oral contraceptives have been shown to lower the levels of six nutrients: riboflavin, B6, folic acid, vitamin B12, ascorbic acid and zinc. Entire books and manuscripts have been written about the health effects of B vitamin deficiency. I simply want to make you aware of this connection so that you may investigate it further.

The main facts on Vitamin B's that are most important:

1. Vitamin B6 must be obtained from the diet because humans cannot synthesize it.
2. B vitamins, especially B6, "play(s) a vital role in the function of approximately 100

enzymes that catalyze essential chemical reactions in the human body"[18]

3. Many studies suggest oral contraception causes B6 depletion; this is detrimental to our health in a number of ways.

4. The binding of PLP (B6) …. "suggests that the vitamin B6 status of an individual may have implications for diseases affected by steroid hormones (such as estrogen and testosterone) including breast cancer and prostate cancers."

5. B6 depletion can inhibit/reduce the production of serotonin, our happy chemical in our brains. This depletion may lead to depression. Depletion of serotonin also increases a woman's risk of developing insomnia and other sleep disorders.

Vitamin C Depletion and the Pill

Estrogen-containing contraceptives (birth control pills) are known to lower vitamin C levels in plasma and white blood cells.[19]

Cholesterol and the Pill

"Birth control pills can affect cholesterol levels. How much of an effect depends on the type of pill you're taking and what concentration of estrogen or progestin it contains. The estrogen in birth control pills causes an increase in high-density lipoprotein (HDL) cholesterol levels (the "good" cholesterol), a decrease in low-density lipoprotein (LDL) cholesterol levels (the "bad" cholesterol) and an increase in your total cholesterol and triglyceride levels. Progestin in birth control pills has the opposite effect."[20]

Acne and the Pill

Authors at the *Cochrane Collaboration* reviewed "combined oral contraceptive (COC's) pills for treatment of acne" and concluded: "The four COCs evaluated in placebo-controlled trials are effective in reducing inflammatory and non-inflammatory facial acne lesions. Few important differences were found between COC types in their effectiveness for treating acne. How COCs compare to alternative acne treatments is unknown since limited data were available regarding this question."[21]

Calcium Deficiency and the Pill
Osteoporosis is a general weakening of your bones and often causes bone fractures later in life.[22] In 2004 *The Journal of Adolescence Health* stated: "Additional findings suggest a potential adverse effect of an OC containing 20 microg ethinyl estradiol/100 microg levonorgestrel on bone health in adolescents."[23]
Peak bone building years are between the ages of 12-22 for young women. Bone density built during these years is crucial to avoid hip fractures as we

age which are one of the most common surgeries in the U.S. for women over 60 years old.

Amenorrhea (no periods) and the Pill
Amenorrhea is the absence of menstruation during the reproductive years. Taking "The Pill" pushes the pause button on ovulation, and for some women, pushing the start button after quitting the pill does not work that easily. Sometimes getting a normal cycle back takes months or even years.

Breast Cancer and the Pill

Recent research implicates the combined estrogen/progestin birth control pills to increased risks for breast cancer.

"In particular, synthetic progesterone derivatives (progestins) such as medroxyprogesterone acetate (MPA), used in millions of women for hormone replacement therapy and contraceptives, markedly increase the risk of developing breast cancer"
www.ncbi.nlm.nih.gov/pubmed/20881962

Please check into this National Institute of Health study called: "Osteoclast differentiation factor RANKL controls development of progestin-driven mammary cancer" from IMBA, Institute of Molecular Biotechnology of the Austrian Academy of Sciences, 1030 Vienna, Austria.

Other references include:

www.imba.oeaw.ac.at/news-media/news/news/osteoclast-differentiation-factor-rankl-controls-development-of-progestin-driven-mammary-cancer/

www.nature.com/nature/journal/v468/n7320/full/nature09387.html

www.foodconsumer.org/newsite/Non-food/Disease/breast_cancer_news_0430130720.html

Your Part 5

Make a list of the pros and con's of using the birth control pill or other form of artifical hormones..
 Birth control is a personal choice and there are many viable options available.

The list of pro's and con's you write today may not fit your life 1 year from now or 5 years from now so remember to re-do this list as your life changes. (you may want to do this on your computer or larger piece of paper this is a really important part of your work. Don't neglect it. This is only for your eyes and heart, known one elses. Getting clear on this issue will help you make the best decisions for your body.

PRO'S	CONS	

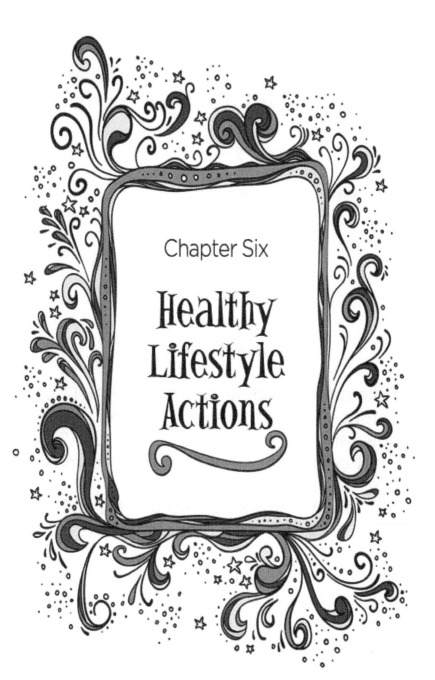

Chapter Six

Healthy Lifestyle Actions

Chapter 6

Healthy Lifestyle Actions

I once heard a spry 92 year old, hunched over man say, "If I knew I was going to live this long I would have taken better care of my body."
What about you?

You are half way through

5 Days left!

Keep Going!

Take a look back at the "YOUR PART" pages before you start this next chapter. See how far you've already come in just 5 days. Start each and every day with this mantra.

" I am taking responsible for my own health and it feels great!"

In this chapter you will read about the "Top Eleven Lifestyle Action Steps" (I tried to keep it to ten but there were just too many).

Each Action Step may seem small on its own, but each will show you how to take better care of your body and take responsibility for YOUR health. What might seem like small changes will add up to HUGE changes. Your hormones will thank you by giving you less mood swings, less brain fog and less fatigue. What will you do first will all this new found energy?

Let's GO!

I have grouped the 11 Action Steps into three categories.

- **Physical Action Steps**
- **Environmental Action Steps**
- **Personal Action Steps**

Let's dive right in!

Physical Action Steps

1. Exercise & Weight Control

Exercise can't be under estimated as a health benefit. Nothing new here, right? The reason you hear about exercise so often is because our lifestyles today are extremely sedentary. We were not made to sit at a desk or a car all day long.[25] The end result of less movement is weight gain. Body fat stores excess hormones and causes mass chaos in our menstrual cycles.

You can find plenty of information on the benefits of exercise just about everywhere today: T.V., radio, Youtube, books etc.. Our sedentary lifestyle is killing us and we have to get off the couch and out of our cars and move our bodies every single day. I will leave information about exercise and weight control changes to the other million books and magazines on the shelves.

I do however recommend jogging and/or walking for everyone; It doesn't cost anything, you can do it everywhere, around the block or at indoor malls regardless if the weather is cooperating. There is simply no excuse not to walk. No matter what your weight, you can start walking. Studies show that walking as little as 30 minutes a day can make a huge difference in your health. Whether you do this or join a gym or an exercise class, you must do something every day.- Once or twice a week is not enough!

I love info graphics and this one is quite clever:
"Sitting Is Killing You"
www.mindbodygreen.com/0-2420/Sitting-Is-Killing-You-Infographic.html

Only One Weight Control Pointer

I do want to make one quick mention of what I consider "junk food" or food with high fructose corn-syrup (HFCS). This needs mentioning because research points to a link between higher estrogen levels in those who consume large quantities of high fructose corn syrup. Nearly ALL processed foods contain high fructose corn syrup. The concern is HFCS is processed in the liver and this may lead to decreased levels of globulin in the liver.   Decreased liver globulin reduces the liver's ability to process the estrogen and consequently the estrogen stays in the blood stream longer and at higher quantities. When this happens it's called circulating estrogen. Too much circulating estrogen all month long leads to estrogen dominance which you read about in Chapter 3. Reducing HFCS will also help you lose weight- yet another reason to look closely at labels and see what you're really eating.

Check out:
www.annieappleseedproject.org/hifrcosylito.html

Simple Movements

During your menstrual cycle when your cramps are at their worst and just getting out of bed seems like too much exercise, here are alternative suggestions for physical movement that will help:

I prefer to call these "movements" rather than "exercises" because most of us can't possibly think about exercise when we are doubled over in pain. All of these movements are designed to be done during your menstrual cycle.

These simple stretches and small movements should be done for at least 10 minutes and you will notice a difference when you finish. You may want to do these more than once a day, depending on your needs. Moving your stagnant energy, also known as Qi in Eastern medicine, is the principle behind this movement concept. You will relieve tension in your abdomen, your back and help increase the blood flow to these areas which helps relieve pain naturally.

Incorporate these movements into your exercise regime and over the next few months you will notice the severity of your period pain will lesson as you build pelvic strength and stamina.

Be A Baby - ahhh feels so good

Directions: Kneel on the floor. Touch your big
toes together and sit on your heels, then separate
your knees about as wide as your hips. Exhale and
lay your torso down between your thighs. Broaden
your sacrum across the back of your pelvis and
narrow your hip points toward the navel, so that
they nestle down onto the inner thighs. Lengthen
your tailbone. Lay your hands on the floor
alongside your torso, palms up, and release the
fronts of your shoulders toward the floor. Feel how
the weight of the front shoulders pulls the shoulder
blades wide across your back. Stay anywhere from
30 seconds to a few minutes.

Be A Bridge   How I spell R-E-L-I-E-F

Directions: Lie on your back and if necessary place
a thickly folded blanket under your shoulders to
protect your neck. Bend your knees and set your
feet on the floor, heels as close to the sitting bones
as possible.

Exhale and press your inner feet and arms actively
into the floor, push your tailbone upward toward
the pubis, firming (but not hardening) the
buttocks, and lift your butt off the floor. Keep your
thighs and inner feet parallel. Clasp the hands
below your pelvis and extend through the arms to
help you stay on the tops of your shoulders. Lift
your butt until the thighs are about parallel to the

floor. Lift your pelvis toward the navel. Keep your shoulder blades pressing firm against the floor. Stay in this pose anywhere from 30 seconds to 1 minute. Release with an exhalation. Repeat 3 times and then reward yourself. You are doing great things for your body your mind and your Period cramps.

Be A Snake   So good for your back!

This rejuvenating movement stimulates both the back and front of the body, especially the lumbar and pelvic regions.

Directions: Lay on your belly with your forehead on the floor. Bend arms at your elbows next to your chest, fingers pointing forward, elbows in. Inhalation, rise up from the forehead, nose, and chin, continuing the stretch through your neck, upper body, and your lower pelvic basis begins tilting upward. Feel the weight shift as you start supporting yourself on your arms. Gradually straighten the arms, broadening your shoulders, stretching and curving your spine, and tightening your buttocks. At the more advanced level your weight can be supported on the tops of your feet and your hands but this is not necessary to get great benefit from this pose. Hold for 30 seconds to one minute.

Remember to avoid practicing inverted poses (no head stands or hand stands) during menstruation.

Slowing down and nurturing yourself at this time of month will make a huge difference even if you do this for just 5-10 minutes a day. Make a habit of doing these and other movements and you will start to reap the rewards.

You don't have to be a Yogi to do these poses, however I encourage you to join a yoga class or start a yoga practice. Research shows that yoga type exercises, meditation and relaxation techniques result in consistent health benefits including a reduction of anxiety and depression.

2. <u>Raw Food Diet & Food Temperatures</u>

Let's talk about food from a different perspective.

First Raw Food

Raw food diets have recently become more popular. A raw food diet consists of unprocessed and uncooked plant foods such as fresh fruit, vegetables, sprouts, seeds, nuts, grains, beans and seaweed. This can be a fairly dramatic dietary change for some. I definitely endorse eating some raw food everyday. But not as a way of life. You'll understand more about this after reading about food temperatures below.

I would recommend however, one raw food day each month. This is a great way to boost your body's natural detox abilities Also a great way to elliminate and reduce re-circulating estrogen.(more about this later in the chapter) Choose any day(s) that works for you. Maybe a weekend is easier than the work/school week. It will help provide the fiber you need to increase bowel movements and avoid the dreaded bloating or constipation that can become prevalent just before bleeding starts.

If you can, choose Day 30 or Day 1 of your cycle to eat raw. This is the day just before your Period starts of the first day of bleeding. If this is not possible don't stress over it. Maybe you are not sure when you're getting your period or the timing just does not work for you, don't worry. Trying a raw food diet is more important than the specific day of the month. Often even a small diet change can make a big difference in the way you feel. You will notice both a physical and emotional change with any major dietary changes. Especially a change away for processed sugary foods..

Raw Food Diet from an Eastern Medicine Perspective:

Traditional Chinese Medicine,(TCM) and Chinese Nutrition classifies all foods by there energetic temperatures. Although this is not common in the West it has been part of Chinese nutrition and disease prevention for centuries. The yin and yang of food preparations and dietary knowledge has been passed down through generations. Eastern medicine considers food the first line of defense against disease. As Hippocrates said, "Let food be thy medicine, and medicine by thy food " Even though Hippocrates was Greek, he had the same philophosy about food, as Chinese traditions.

 Entire books have been written on food classifications from a Chinese nutrition perspective and you can find these suggestions in the References section of this book. Here is a brief explanation of how Eastern medicine uses food to complement an individual's constitution, and how it can help you STOP YOUR BITCHING & put an end to your menstrual cramps.

Cold Food

In Traditional Chinese Nutrition and TCM, cold foods have a cooling effect in your body. These foods are not necessarily eaten straight out of a refrigerator or freezer, but rather foods that have inherent properties of cooling the body's heat energy or the yang energy A diet which includes cold foods during the summer time is preferrable not during the winter. Eating an abundance of cold foods for a prolonged time can interfere with your menstrual cycle which is why this is an important discussion for this book. Keeping a balance in temperatures of the foods you eat is the key.

Over consumption of cold foods makes the body work harder to stay warm internally. This may slow digestion and also create a symptom known as "cold uterus" in TCM. (This symptom is discussed in greater detail in Chap. 9) Cold foods are generally fine to eat as long as they are balanced with hot or warm foods. TCM always strives to balance the body and this includes balancing our diets. A balanced diet of warm, cool, cold, neutral and hot foods is the goal.

Food temperatures are important to consider along with the season and region which you live. Someone living in a hot environment will generally need slightly more cooling foods than someone living in a cold environment. Be sensible about balancing your foods with your climate all year long. Examples of cold foods are: bananas, grape fruit, watermelon, pear, cantaloupe, pork, snow peas, seaweed, clams, salt and white sugar.

Cool Foods

TCM also categorizes some foods as "cool foods". These are not quite as cold as the cold category, but could still deplete the warm, yang energy of the body if eaten in excess. Again the idea is to eat a variety of foods at all times. Women with irregular Periods are advised to eat only moderate amounts of cold/cool foods, especially during cold winter months. Examples of cool foods are: apples, tomatoes, strawberries, cucumbers, tomatoes, spinach, zucchini, dandelion greens, eggplant, broccoli, carrots, eggs, mint, and cilantro. These are only a few commno food examples not a comprehensive listing.

Neutral Foods

Neutral temperature foods have no pronounced effect on internal body temperature, however they are often high in natural sugars and may interfere with insulin production. The ultmate goal is to eat a variety of foods including a moderate amount of all temperatures and types, grains, proteins, carbohydrates, fruits and vegetables. Notice there is not a category for processed (junk) food. Examples of some neutral foods are: celery, beets, honey, rice, bread, sunflower seeds, almonds, yams, lettuce and brown rice.

Warm Foods

Warm foods, you guessed it, have a warming effect on the body. You have probably experience this after eating a spicy bowl of chili that produced a little sweat on your forehead. Warm foods are important for the female body and are often lacking in the Western diet. Warm foods can help maintain the right internal temperature to prevent a cold uterus, which ultimately results in increased cramping and pain. Just to clarify, there is no perfect translation of "cold uterus" in Western medicine terms. But someone who is cold often, has a pale tongue color, eats a lot of salads, drinks a lot of cold drinks will often be diagnoised with cold uterus. This is just one example. Now, eat some warm foods which help increase your internal body temperature. Examples of warm foods are: green and black tea, chives, leeks, peaches, cherries, raspberries, chicken, beef, turkey, ginger, dang gui, rice vinegar, wine, black beans, walnuts and coffee.

Hot Foods

Hot foods are not necessarily spicy foods. Hot foods increase blood flow including the blood flow to the internal organs. Hot foods are also very good for increasing the immune system and fighting off free radicals. Examples of hot foods are: garlic, scallions, black pepper, lamb, cinnamon and dry ginger. Overeating hot foods can lead to hormone imbalance so be careful to eat these foods with a combination of other temperature foods.

Eating too many salads, cold drinks, ice cream, frozen yogurt and other foods outlined in the cold and cool sections above can hamper your efforts to have pain free, bitch free Periods.

I highly recommend cutting out ice cold beverages in favor of room temperature or warm drinks until you've gotten the PMS and cramps under control.

What's most important is to eat a variety of different temperature foods in any single day. The week before your Period, you could focus on adding some of these foods; green onions, spinach, walnuts, cinnamon, Chinese dates, fennel, black pepper and ginger to your diet.

Eat meat, fruits and processed sugar in moderation (no more than 10% of your daily food intake). This is not a diet, but an overall philosophy of eating. Reducing consumption of cold foods, alcohol, caffeine, sugar and dairy especially the week before your Period will help. Commit to your goal of a better you, and make food choices that will really help YOU be a better YOU!

FOR Healthy Food Suggestions Go to the back section of this book called Suggestions for Food Choices.

Also Check out this graphic on sugar consumption.

www.onlinenursingprograms.com/nursing-your-sweet-tooth/

3. **Stay Hydrated - H2O Update**

The best way to stay hydrated is to drink plenty of water throughout the day. Water is the essential fluid of life. If you wait until you get thirsty, you've deprived your body of essential minerals and make your body work much harder to stay in a state of homeostasis or balance. Our body always strives for fluid and mineral balance. Experts agree our bodies needs 6 - 8 ounce glasses of water a day. I would add this varies depending on the outside temperature and your exertion level. Alcohol, tea and caffeinated beverages do not count as water. Soft drinks definitely do not count. Soft drinks are empty calories full of sugar and chemicals with absolutely no health benefits. Six glasses of water each day is your goal (try adding a little fresh lemon). This will improve your mental clarity and give your taste buds a little something more to think about. Additionally, lemon helps your body keep its acid/alkaline balance in check.

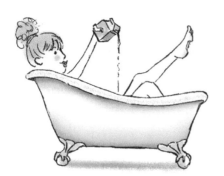

Another way to stay hydrated is to soak in an Epsom salt bath. The natural mineral in the salts will be absorbed through your skin and your body only takes what it needs.

A warm water bath will also alleviate cramps during your cycle.

Epsom salt can be found in small bags or milk carton type containers at just about any pharmacy. This is a "my grandmother use to do that" kind of recommendation,m unfortunately often overlooked today. These old fashioned remedies have value, so give it a try.

By the way, soaking in a bath does not necessarily have to be a time consuming event. I often hear, from my patients, "I don't have time for a bath!" I have to be at work, school, etc. Here's how to fit a bath into your busy schedule. Fill the tub with 4 inches of hot to warm water, this only takes 5 minutes. Dissolve some epsom salts and get in. Sponge water on the areas of your body not submerged. Lay there for 5 minutes. Your bath now took the same amount of time as a shower and you probably used less water. Even just 5 minutes of relaxing in warm water will make a huge difference. You will feel relaxed and your body will be fully hydrated, this also improves your cognitive thinking skills. You will feel clear headed and this is a great way to start your day!

4. <u>Acne Solution- One Thing Is Clear</u>

Since I'm talking about healthy life style actions I wanted to include an acne solution. Often times girls/women use "The Pill" to reduce acne. There are much safer and more effective treatments for acne and this herbal remedy happens to be one of those. Not only is it herbal, but it has excellent research substantiating its effectiveness.

Thyme (yes, thyme the same spice you might cook with) used in a tincture can be as effective as acne lotions according to recent research. A study of herbal preparations conducted at Leeds Metropolitan found that thyme tincture has the greatest antibacterial effect. In fact, thyme was better than the active ingredients in most acne creams and washes such as benzoyl peroxide.

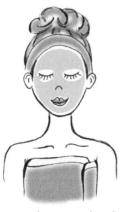 This is fantastic news for those who suffer with acne and spend thousands of dollars on prescription creams and washes. The study was presented at the Society for General Microbiology's Conference in March 2012. A thyme tincture is much gentler than many of the harsh chemicals in acne creams and washes and can be applied with a cotton ball several times a day

You can find this acne solution here:

shop.pacherbs.com/Herbal-Acne-Treatment-Naturally-Cure-Acne-With-Thyme-Pacific-Herbs

5. **Heating Pads**

Heating pads are an easy option to relieve pain anytime during your Period. There is absolutely no downside to (non-electrical) heating pads. The old fashioned hot water bottle worked for grandma and can work for you too. If you're going to use a heating bad try the ones that heat up in a micro-wave oven rather than the plug-in, electrical type. You decide what works for you.

I also recommend the more mobile version of the heating pad: the stick on the skin heating patches that are sold in many stores today. These are great when you're on the go but need some relief, especially for your back. Check out this link for the herbal ones that work great for hours.
 shop.pacherbs.com/pain-terminator-patch-Golden-Sunshine

6. **Cleansing - Douching**

Women throughout time have found cleansing their vagina an important routine for spiritual and physical health. Douching can be a simple 50% warm water /50% vinegar solution. I prefer apple cider vinegar over white vinegar, but either one works. If you prefer, get a premade store-bought douche. Douching is best done on a toilet/bidet or in the shower. Tub douching is not recommended as you do not want to soak in the same water that is being expunged. Some women prefer douching on the first day of their cycle and find cleaning out some blood can bring some relief. However, the uterus rarely sheds all its blood in a few minutes or hours.

Douching can remove normal vaginal flora otherwise known as the healthy bacteria. For this reason, I don't recommend it more than every two weeks for healthy women. For some women, douching can relieve cramps at the onset of menstruation or at the end of your cycle. This is a personal choice that may or may not be an enjoyable cleansing process for you.

See more information here on "Vaginal Douching: Evidence for Risks or Benefits to Women's Health" http://epirev.oxfordjournals.org/content/24/2/109.full

7. <u>Daily Bowel Movement</u>

This is one of the most important questions Oriental Medicine Doctors also known as Licensed Acupuncturists in the U.S.A. may ask.

I can't stress enough how important it is to have healthy bowel movements (BM) throughout your life. Many of us overlook this because it's not terribly glamorous to talk about. A daily bowel movement ensures we are not reabsorbing and re-circulating excess hormones. The body works best when toxins are excreated daily and BM's are one way the body elliminates toxins. We don't need additional estrogen circulating in our blood stream when the body has already sent it to the colon and it is being processed for ellimination.

A healthy colon is imperative to good health. In relation to our discussion on PMS, and mestrual cramps this is an important topic and sometimes overlooked in Western medicine. Our bodies are designed to make and dispose of estrogen, progesterone and other hormones. It is your job to make sure this occurs everyday.

Remember, our bodies are always changing and this is another aspect of this change. Our bodies inherently have fluctuating hormone levels from day to day and week to week. If we don't dispose of the excess hormones or unneeded waste, it can build up and wreak havoc by being reabsorbed and transported back through the body.

A *daily* bowel movement is one healthy habit you absolutely must not overlook. Unfortunately, many of us rush around and are not always in a convenient location "to go". Making sure you have time in the morning (an excellent time for a BM) before running off to school or work is one way to encourage BM. As discussed above, staying hydrated will also make a difference in your ability to have a BM. Be sure to drink enough water all day long. Some people have more than one BM daily and that is certainly fine as long as it is a formed stool and not diarrhea. Your goal is at least one formed BM daily.

A high fat and refined sugar diet lacking in fiber will effect your daily BM. Fiber is what gives your large intestine the bulk it needs to form a stool. Eating enough fiber is key to healthy bowel movements. If you don't currently have a BM daily, then add high fiber cereals, legumes (beans), seeds, nuts, and veggies like celery to your daily food intake. Our daily intake of food each day must coincide with daily out-take, otherwise known as poop. Alcohol, antibiotics, antacids and over the counter pain relievers can also contribute to poor bowel health. Limiting these will help you maintain healthy colon habits for life.

A couple of tips I give my patients to increase bowel movements if and when your bowels get sluggish are:
- eat a couple dry prunes daily
- drink a cup of prune juice daily
- add aloe vera juice daily
- add fiber to your diet like raw carrots and celery snacks
- Add seeds like chia, hemp, walnuts, sesame and flax seeds, which all contain natural oils that help your colon stay healthy

- I also recommend herbal remedies and hydration to increase BM's

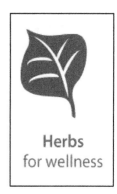

Herbs
for wellness

Remember, bowel movements can become especially difficult a day or two before your Period starts so pay particular attention to the foods you're eating and the habits you're keeping during these days.When we feel good, we are all a lot less bitchy.

Environmental Action Steps

Hair Nail & Cosmetics Products

*Your skin is an organ, what you put **ON** your body affects your health!*

Compared to men, women use at least 10-15 more products for their skin, face, hair and nails each day. These products can have more effects on your body than meets the eye. Cosmetics, hair and nail products deserve a quick mention because the amount of harmful chemicals in them can have unexpected effects on our hormone balance and overall body chemistry. Many contain chemicals that make your hormones go haywire and many have now been proven to cause cancer.

Hair products cosmetics and even products we use to clean our homes contain ingredients that are toxic and can and throw our hormones out of whack. The Campaign for Safe Cosmetics (CSC), a nonprofit advocacy group based in San Francisco and financed in part by the Breast Cancer Fund, a nonprofit organization says, people are exposed to roughly 126 different chemicals daily, many of which have not been thoroughly tested.

Research the products you purchase and especially those you use on your skin. You may not have realized the impact they can have on your health. Ladies, please realize the power of purchasing!! When you purchase from companies that list long chemical names that we can't possibly understand, then your dollars are supporting the toxic chemical industry.

Please use only pure organic skin and hair products or don't buy them at all. Make your own when possible. Also, do a little research on the makeup you use daily. Consider the big picture here: Years of exposure to these chemicals and toxic metals does damage to your cells that is not repairable.

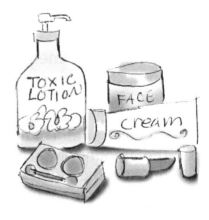

I know, organic products are a little more expensive, but isn't your health worth it? At the bare minimum choose paraben-free versions of nonorganic products. Better yet, DIY and make your own soaps, shampoos even toothpaste.

The skin is the body's largest organ. Our skin is porous, allowing us to sweat and allowing us to absorb what's applied to it. Treat your skin and entire outer body with the same care you treat your inner body. Lipstick with lead should not be applied, and shampoos with parabens should not be used on your hair. Remember: your body is YOUR temple so treat it like one. You can be clean, green and frugal by making your own homemade beauty products. Google "homemade cosmetics" for more than 400,000 pages of recipes and instructions.

Lisa Archer, the national coordinator for The Campaign for Safe Cosmetic's CSC, has this to say about cosmetics:

"The system for regulating cosmetics in the U.S. is virtually nonexistent. Other countries are far ahead. The E.U., European Union for example, has banned the use of more than 1,000 substances in cosmetics; in contrast, the FDA has banned the use of eight substances for use in cosmetics."

Parabens are one of the top offenders. You must eliminate these to help you normalize your menstrual cycles and end PMS.

Parabens are synthetic estrogens! This means they act like estrogen in your body and disrupt your hormone system. This is exactly what we need to prevent to end PMS and Stop Our Bitching! Some studies show parabens have a link to breast cancer. A 2004 study found parabens in breast cancer tumors from 19 of 20 women studied. According to the Breast Cancer Fund, six different parabens have been identified in breast cancer tumors.
A 2006 Center for Disease Control study found parabens in nearly all urine samples from a demographically diverse sample of U.S. adults. This indicates widespread exposure of parabens in the U.S. population. The European Union banned the use of sodium methylparaben in fragrance due to its ability to strip skin of pigment and other health concerns.Read the ingredient label looking for "-paraben" or "parabens".

You may see it under these names:

methylparaben, propylparaben, butylparapen and ethylparaben.

Some products are beginning to advertise that they are "paraben- free" on the label so look for these.

What about nano-particles?

Nano-Particles are little tiny particles, so small that when put them on our skin they can enter our red blood cells. Cosmetic companies have been using this miniaturizing technology for nearly a decade. They turn ingredients into nano-particles that are invisible to the naked eye. Shrinking ingredients makes products a more desirable consistency and eases application. The perfect example is the use of zinc oxide as nano-particles in sunscreens. Nano technology elliminates that "chalk white" effect you get on your skin when the sun screen doesn't rub in completely. Companies didn't like the complaints from consumer and nano technology has now created sun screen that disappers quickly when applied to your skin. Except, nobody is telling you these nano particles are easily absorbed into your blood stream.

So What's The Problem?

Minerals like titanium dioxide and zinc oxide are commonly found in sunscreen lotions, foundation and other liquid types of lotions were not as dangerous sitting on the skin. They were less harmful in their normal size (these chemicals were too large to penetrate the protective layers of your skin). However, as nanoparticles they absorb into your skin since they are smaller than a red blood cell.

Research shows that nano-particles of zinc oxide and other ingredients like aluminum collect in the brain and cause cell death. Nano-particles are so easily absorbed that they can be detectable in all areas of the body, including vital organs. Damage occurs with frequency of use because higher concentrations increase toxicity.

Now that you know the dangers, use your makeup money to say "Hell No" to the status quo. Don't buy from companies that don't list their ingredients. Email these companies and tell them why you won't use their products and shop for makeup at a health food store you can trust.

IF YOUR COSMETICS DON'T LIST INGREDIENTS – TOSS THEM IN THE GARBAGE!!

Manufacturers will stop making chemical laden cosmetics when we stop buying them. Support the makers of wholesome products, big and small. The world will be a better place when you and everyone else start really speaking up with the dollars you spend. Forget the advertising, it's there to convince you their product is something you need and want. Make up your own mind. Can you live without it? Can you use something healthier? When you're shopping ask yourself these questions.

When you buy cosmetics or any personal care product, buy it from a trusted source and ALWAYS **Read the Labels!**

Check out this compelling story from a young woman with thyroid cancer, and why she say's we need safer products:

http://blog.saferchemicals.org/2012/08/im-32-and-battling-cancer.html#.UC0olv8ufFQ.facebook

I often shop at my local health food store and they do the research for me.   I know the cosmetic products they carry are safe and chemical free. This saves me from reading all those labels full of chemical names I can't pronounce.

To see if your lipstick or other cosmetic products made the FDA UNSAFE list, take a look at these two sites.

http://www.fda.gov/Cosmetics/ProductandIngredientSafety/Product Information/

www.fda.gov/Safety/MedWatch/SafetyInformation

Also check out the Environmental Working Group (EWG) website where you can search almost any personal care product. See exactly if your skin, hair and nail product ingredients are safe or dangerous based on the EWG's extensive research and ratings.

Skin Deep Cosmetic Safety Database is another helpful site in finding and evaluating healthful, green products:
http://www.cosmeticsdatabase.com/index.php?nothanks=1

A word on Phthalates

Phthalates, more chemicals, appear on product labels often in disguise under the names:

Vinyl, PVC, phthalates, DEHP, DBP, fragrance, parfum

Their effects on us are similar to parabens; phthalates are endo-disrupting and hormone disrupting chemicals.

Endo-disrupting chemicals have been linked to obesity. A 2008 study by the Environmental Working Group detected 7 out of 7 phthalates in all 20 of the 20 teen girls tested. Phthalates are not regulated by the U.S. federal government.
In 2004, the European Union banned thousands of bibutyl phthalate (DBP) and diethylhexyl phthalate (DEHP) from personal care products. The state of California placed DEHP on its Prop 65 list of chemicals known to cause cancer and reproductive toxicity. Phthalates are also used to make plastics soft and flexible.

A 2002 study tested 72 cosmetic products from major U.S. brands and found phthalates in nearly

75% of them. None of them had the word phthalates on the label. (Learning this puts me in a really bitchy mood, how about you?).

Reduce Your Exposure to Phthalates:

- Avoid Vinyl and PVC plastic. Unless the manufacture specifies the product is phthalate-free, avoid soft vinyl products with a strong plastic smell including toys and shower curtains. Choose fabric or non-plastic cosmetic bags.
- Look for #3 on plastics products, food containers or bottles. #3 = phthalates
- Check cosmetics: shampoos and conditioners, lotions, perfumes, nail polish, hair spray
- Check vinyl products, including friendly looking rubber duckies
- Check products containing "fragrance"
- Even check plastic clothing like raincoats and rainboots.
- Some plastic food containers contain phthalates
- Read the labels and look for "phthalate-free" cosmetics.
- Avoid products with fragrance. Phthalates are used in "fragrance" mixtures that are added to cosmetic products.

Names you should look for:
and It's all greek to me..

I think the better rule is if you can't understand the word and it doesn't sound like english... you should probably stay away from it.

Phthalates can appear on labels in many forms: DEHP, butyl benzyl phthalate, di-n-butyl phthalate, di-n-octyl phthalate, diethyl phthalate dimethyl phthalate, mono- (2-ethyl-5-hydroxyhexyl), mono- (2-ethyl-5-oxohexyl), mono-2-ethylhexyl phthalate, mono-butyl phthalate, monobenzyl phthalate, monoethyl phthalate, monomethyl phthalate.

You may also want to check out research from *The Journal of Environmental Health Perspectives* on phthalates linked to diabetes.

Simple Ways To Stop Your Bitching

& Be Chemical FREE

1. **Transparency, Transparency, Transparency. Look for products that list ingredients.**

2. **Check out the Campaign for Safe Cosmetics -Champions for some of the best manufacturers.**

3. **Look for certifications which are now on some safe, chemical free beauty products.**

4. **Choose brands that have earned NPA Natural, USDA Organic, NSF/ANSI "contains organic," NaTrue or EcoCert labels, all of which prohibit the use of phthalates.**

5. **Shop at stores you trust.**

Many natural products retailers enforce their own ingredient standards. Be a good conscious consumer and support only companies that support your health.

NOW THAT YOU'RE CHEMICAL FREE ON THE OUTSIDE...
Let's talk about chemicals you may be adding to the inside of your body that are making you bitchy.

What are BPA's?

BPA, or Bisphenol A, is an EDC (Endocrine Disrupting Chemical) found in plastic water bottles and lurking in other places discussed below. First, let's look at the water bottles. Bisphenol A (BPA) on the label you will see:

Polycarbonate Plastics

Bottles such as nalgene polycarbonate are popular for drinking water bottles. However, polycarbonate (plastic) releases this chemical known as BPA. The plastic industry safety studies have denied any significant health effects from one time use plastic water bottles for years, yet 90% of government studies found harmful health effects. These effects are magnified in young children and expecting moms and may also affect male sexuality and reproduction. But times are a changing and BPA's are now being outlawed in baby bottles.

Why are BPA's dangerous?

The problem is that bisphenol-A acts as a "xeno-estrogen." This means it acts like the female hormone estrogen in our bodies. But of course, it's not our real estrogen, it is a "stranger" to the body. This was discussed in Chapters 2 & 3. Breast cancer risk is increased in women who carry higher amounts of xeno-estrogens, and both men and women are subject to a huge range of other harmful health effects. The most far-reaching effects are birth defects and miscarriages. Another harmful effect is the disruption of beta cell function in the pancreas, which creates a pre-diabetes type condition of high blood insulin and insulin resistance.

The CDC data shows that 93% of 2,157 people tested, between the ages of six and 85, had detectable levels of BPA's by-product in their urine. "Children had higher levels than adolescents and adolescents had higher levels than adults," says endocrinologist Retha Newbold of the U.S. National Institute of Environmental Health Sciences, who found that BPA impairs fertility in female mice. "In animals, BPA can cause permanent effects after very short periods of exposure. It doesn't have to remain in the body to have an effect."

The first and absolutely essential habit you must change is to stop drinking any water out of disposable plastic water bottles. Drink water out of glass or a BPA Free plastic bottle you can refill yourself.

Another change, a simply one that you might already be doing is washing your hands, especially before eating and certainly after touching cash register receipts. The reason is simple. Cash register receipts are made from a thermal paper that contains high amounts of BPA's. When you touch these receipts or even handle cash today (much of the BPA's are landing on our cash), you can potentially have even higher amounts of BPA's on your hands. This is so easy and even though may seem like a minor thing to do in the scheme of things, it is actually quite important. Wash your hands before you eat and after you touch thermal receipts. Make this a daily habit.

Often times we eat on the run, pick up fast food and have just touched the receipt of the food we bought. It is simple to politely decline taking a store receipt if you don't need it. New research has even found BPS a similar toxic chemical to BPA's on 87% of our everyday cash throughout the United States.

Alternatives to BPA's are being developed even as this book goes to print. Unfortunately, we really don't know if those alternatives are any safer than BPA's since newer chemicals haven't really been tested either. PVC, which is full of pthalates, is one "alternative" to BPA. There is some suggestion that bisphenol S (BPS), a BPA alternative, might have even more estrogenic activity. I don't know if that will turn out to be true, but these alternatives do require more testing.

Canned food is another place where high concentrations of BPA's are found. Crazy but true. Pressure is mounting on some canned food manufacturers and they are looking for alternatives and are in the beginning stages of phasing out BPA's in the lining of cans. Canned tomatoes or tomato sauce in the can is one of the worst offenders. The natural acidic nature of tomatoes seems to breakdown the BPA lining in the can and become concentrated in the tomatoes. If you eat a lot of canned tomatoes, switch to buying them in glass jars or cardboard milk type containers.

"Healthy Child Healthy World" has a campaign to remove BPA's from our food supply. Help them out and visit their website:
www.healthychild.org/main/

The FDA recently (finally) banned BPA's in baby bottles, whereas Canada had banned the sale of BPA baby bottles years earlier.

Summary to reduce your exposure to BPA's:

For more information:
Environmental Defense BPA fact sheet
Government of Canada's BPA fact sheet
CDC's report of U.S. residents exposure to BPA

Watch a great video on BPA's at
www.youtube.com/watch?feature=player_embedded&v=N3_cYZKksvI

My motto: .

I like my hormones on a short leash

and house broken.

In other words... I want as much control as possible. I don't need hormones running amuck all over the place. They make a mess of my neurotransmitters which put me on an emotional rollercoaster. If you've ever felt this way, you know what I mean.

Feel free to use my motto if you can relate to it. If you know a product has chemicals in it that can cause hormonal imbalance, why would you want to use it? Isn't the goal to STOP YOUR BITCHING?

If your hormones are running the show, then you will be bitchy... guaranteed.

Last Chemical In The List...I Promise!

One last chemical to avoid like the plague: Triclosan - "antibacterial" soaps. It might seem harmless, but this is another endocrine disrupting chemical and you don't want it on your hands or anywhere on your body. By now you've heard this so many times: Even in small amounts (even at 1 part per billion), endocrine disrupting hormones mess with your menstrual cycle, throw off your thyroid functions and mess with your delicately balanced hormones.

Triclosan was found in 20 of 20 teens girls tested in an Environmental Working Group 2008 study on chemicals in teen bodies. (Triclosan also may degrade into a type of dioxin, a hazardous toxin.)

A FDA advisory panel concluded that "antibacterial" soaps, including those with triclosan, are no better than regular soap and water at killing germs or reducing infections.

As you reduce your exposure to these chemicals, you will start seeing a difference in your body's hormonal fluctuations and you will more easily put your body back into a balanced state all month long. Baby steps here will add up. So keep at it!!

Check your products for triclosan it's commonly found in:

Antibacterial body care products
mattresses, pillows
textiles, underwear and socks
soap
face and body washes
acne treatment
lotions
detergents
toothpastes
dishwashing detergent
deodorant
creams
pesticides

Check the label, triclosan will be listed in the active ingredients. Instead of using antibacterial soap, wash your hands with normal soap and warm water for 15-20 seconds. If you use skin disinfectant, use an alcohol rub or rinse.

Avoid "antibacterial" dishwashing and cleaning products.

Avoid products that say "protection against mold", "odor fighting", or keeps food fresher, longer." These claims may indicate the presence of triclosan.

More resources for you to do your own research:

Environrmental Working Group: Download their APP's to help you while shopping.

www.ewg.org/foodnews/guide/

OR go to the Envirornmental Working Group.website and ask, what is triclosan?

www.ewg.org/node/26721

Now that we've talked about all the chemical toxins you are putting on your skin if you want to know where toxins could be lurking around your house go to this link. www.everydayexposures.com/

Cleaning Products and Laundry

Should we be concerned about laundry detergent and cleaning products? What does this have to do with Period cramps and PMS? A LOT!

Many chemicals in laundry detergents and household cleaning products are not safe to breathe or to have next to your skin. To say there has been a lack of disclosure regarding these chemicals is an understatement. Labels on laundry detergents and household cleaning products are pretty much non-existent.

If you were to learn these products have known cancer causing chemicals, would you want to buy them? I'm sure more consumers would choose the organic versions, if this information was readily available. One chemical called 1,4-Dioxane is present in many commonly used laundry detergents as a **contaminant,** therefore current regulations say it **DOES NOT** have to be disclosed because manufacturers are not intentionally including it in their products.
WHAT? I'm trying my best not to be confusing, but even I'm confused.

Why take chances with these chemicals? I prefer clean clothes with no unnecessary chemical contaminants next to my skin. I can clean my house just fine with all the organic products on the market today along with vinegar, water and baking soda.

You can find lots of research on chemicals in your household items at this link: www.breastcancerfund.org

W

When chemicals affect your endocrine system they affect your hormonal balance. These chemicals have a BITCH factor built in and that's why we want to avoid them.

There are fantastic options today!! You will still have clean clothes and you will not be putting known cancer causing chemicals next to your skin or into the waste water. This is a win–win for you and your environment. The additional cost is nominal. Remember, it's not just the daily exposure to cancer causing chemicals, it is the buildup of these chemicals over years. The

cancer you get at age 50 may be a result of the toxicity levels building throughout your 50 years. The more chemicals you can intentionally avoid when you're young, the better off you'll be at 50, 60, and 70 years old.

Personal Action Plans

Meditation

Everyone can meditate and everyone can benefit. Meditation was once something only hippies did in the 1960's. Today, every magazine, radio station and gym tout the benefits of this ancient practice. I encourage you to spend some time each day in meditation. Simply sit quietly, concentrate on your breathing and clear your mind. It can be as short as 5 minutes but you'll find the longer you practice the more benefits you will reap. Even gardening and doing dishes can be very meditative when there are no distractions.

However, the best way to meditate is to just sit quietly. Whether you are in your bedroom, office, or outdoors, do this for 5-15 minutes each day. It's like a power nap without falling asleep. There are even phone app's now that have a gong sound you can set for 5 min, 10 min etc.; turn it on and get in touch with yourself.

When you meditate, or just sit quietly, you will begin listening to your body. Reduction in anxiety and stress are immediate benefits. Over time you will develop a sense of relaxation that brings clarity. How does this help menstrual cramps?

When you learn how to relax and release tension, even for just a few minutes each day while you're not experiencing pain, you will be able to practice the same techniques when you do have pain. Learning how to release stress will help your Period pain immensely.

Mediations help you tap into your inner pilot light! You can do them anywhere you can be at peace for at least 5 minutes.

Oprah on Meditation

www.mindbodygreen.com/0-3640/Oprah-on-Meditation-It-Makes-Me-1000-Better.htm

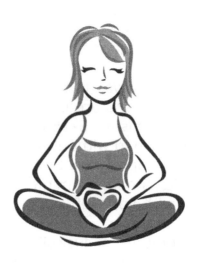

Yoga and Tai Qi

If you have never done yoga or tai qi you have got to try it!! Meditation and deep breathing exercises are both intertwined into yoga and Tai Qi. Both of these movement therapies have tremendous physical, mental and emotional benefits.

Yoga studios have exploded across the country in the last few years. It's a well known mood booster and if you've ever taken a class you know how good you feel when you are finished. Grab a yoga video, find one on the internet or get yourself into a neighborhood yoga studio. It's the easiest exercise to start. Anyone can do it, regardless of age, weight or athletic ability. Do yoga stretches and small movements for at least 10 minutes daily and you will notice a difference. You may want to do these more than once a day, depending on your needs. Moving your stagnant energy, also known as Qi in eastern medicine, is the principal behind this movement concept. You will relieve tension in your abdomen and your back by increasing blood flow to these areas which helps relieve pain naturally.

The goal is the long term reduction and elimination of painful periods, so incorporate these movements into your exercise regimen and over the next few months you will notice the severity of pain will lessen as you build pelvic strength and stamina.
http://nccam.nih.gov/health/tips/yoga?nav=fb

Tai Qi

Tai Qi is another excellent form of movement that anyone at any age can learn. This ancient practice of movement/breathing exercise is easy to learn. Once you've taken a basic beginner class you can practice on your own anywhere, any time. Tai Qi has been passed down throughout Asian cultures and if you visit any Asian community across the U.S. you'll find parks filled with people practicing Tai Qi exercises in the morning. I happened upon such a park one early weekend morning. It was so full of people, the overflow crowd was practicing across the street and even around the corner. But all the participants were following the same routine and the same movements of a leader in one section of the park. It was an amazing sight. Any consistent exercise can help balance your hormones and in the end it's that balance that will create a healthier you. You can learn some basic Tai Chi on Youtube, but a class is really your best bet for learning this ancient art.

Your Part 6

Make it your resolution, your job and your goal to try something new. This chapter has an overwhelming amount of information and you may want to go back and read it over next month. Maybe you can't do everything in this chapter right away, but of the 11 major action steps you can start with 1 or 2 and start making small changes. If you already do a few of the things listed in this Chapter, pick a new habit to change.

Maybe you don't drink from plastic water bottles so you get a gold star for already doing that action step. Your job for this chapter is choosing and starting at least one new thing. Write that first thing here!

My new healthy action this month will be

_____Date_____

Begin limiting the toxic endocrine disrupting chemicals in the products you purchase, start an exercise program or daily meditating, add the movements into your Period days and/or change

up your diet or maybe try out a 24 hour raw food diet. In a month you need to document how you've done on keeping this promise to yourself. So no cheating yourself from the benefits of these activities. You know what they say...
No pain... No gain.

Be honest with yourself! In as little as 30 minutes a day you can make a major change in your body that leaves you feeling fantastic. The fantastic feeling comes from balanced hormones all month long. Once you start feeling this month after month, you will want to add another new healthy action step into your life every month.

You won't want to stop at just one or two changes. Start feeling this today.

Choose a new challenge for your 2nd month. Challenge yourself to keep trying a new action each month going forward.

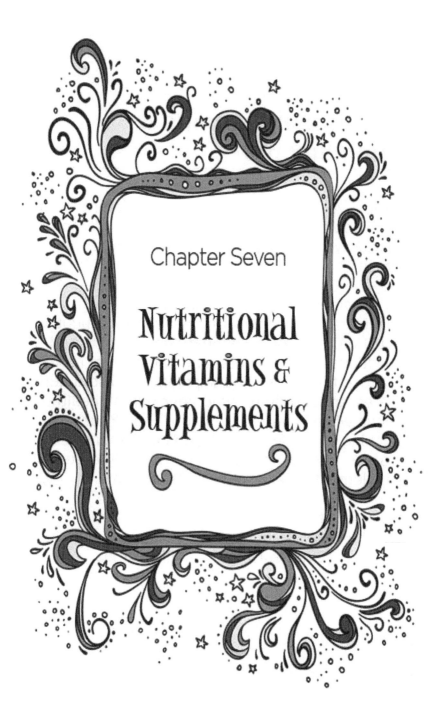

Chapter Seven

Nutritional Vitamins & Supplements

Chapter 7

Nutritional Vitamins & Supplements

I know you've probably heard of different vitamins and supplements to help reduce your cramps, but how do you really know what works and what doesn't?

As a trained health professional, I've spent a considerable number of hours learning about nutrition, attending seminars on vitamins and nutritional supplements, and using them in my practice for years. The supplements listed here are essential to improving your overall health. These will absolutely help you "Stop Your Bitching". These will reduce PMS & menstrual cramps. I'm giving you the absolutely essential supplements you really cannot ignore.

Let's get started.
Which vitamins should I take and what will they do for me? (I've heard this a million times.)

Let's start with B Vitamins

Vitamin B6 is great for bloating and water retention, but a well rounded multi-vitamin high in the B-vitamins is definitely a good place to start. You must take a minimum of 100 to 200 mg daily to make a difference in your menstrual pain. Make this part of your daily routine and you will notice the results even the first month. If you've taken OC (birth control pills) you may need even higher dosages to begin building back B vitamins lost since Vitamin B2, Vitamin B6, Vitamin B12 and Folic Acid are all depleted when taking OC.

Vitamin C

Vitamin C helps combat stress, and you need to take at least 1000 mg daily. (You can get that in 1 pill so this is really not difficult.) A good quality multi-vitamin will probably have 500 mg of Vitamin C but you need closer to 1000 or 1500 mg during stressful times. If you are not getting five servings of fruits and fresh vegetables each day then Vitamin C needs to come in the form of a supplement, period. I prefer vitamin supplelments derived from whole foods there are a few very good brands available.

Vitamin E

Vitamin E is an antioxidant, meaning it protects cell membranes and other fat-soluble parts of the body from damage. Vitamin E is helpful in blocking the formation of prostaglandins, those chemical messengers in your uterus that cause cramping and pain. (Remember, these were discussed in Chapter 3). You can find vitamin E in wheat germ oil, nuts and seeds, whole grains, egg yolks, and vegetables. To help prevent severe menstrual pain, take 400 IU of vitamin E a day starting two days before your period and continue for the first 3 days of bleeding. Five days a month of this supplement is usually enough. Whenever possible, remember it is always better to get your Vitamin E from food sources.[26]

Primrose Oil or Black Current Seed Oil

Although primrose oil and black current seed oil have been touted as natural treatments for PMS and menstrual irregularities, there exists no solid clinical evidence to support these claims.[27] But, if you insist on buy it, try to purchase it in a gel cap form. This packaging prevents natural oxidation of the oils' beneficial omega-6 fatty acids that are essential for many bodily functions. Primrose oil is an excellent source of GLA (gamma-linolenic acid) and a good source of omega 3 fatty acids. (See below) Keep in mind, packaging and processing does effect these oils and they may not be in the same natural and organic state, and therefore not as beneficial, as they would be when consumed naturally in foods.

PMS sufferers have reported feeling much better in studies using evening primrose oil, however there is not much research on this. In the August 1990 issue of *The Medical Journal of Australia*, researchers reported a more careful approach: They divided 38 women in two groups. One took primrose oil and one took a placebo, but both groups reported the same improvement.

Omega 3 Fatty Acids

Omega 3 Fatty Acids (Omega 3's) are another very essential fatty acid and may play a role in reducing depression and relieving symptoms of painful Periods during adolescents. Omega 3's are found in fish or fish oil tablets. According to one study, taking a good quality omega 3 fatty acid supplement containing 1800 mg a day of EPA & DHA for a minimum of two months can benefit menstrual pain.[28] Fish oils can also help regulate how much prostaglandin hormone your cells crank out each month. The less prostaglandins, the less contractility of the uterine and other smooth muscles. Bottom line here: less pain equals less bitching. Always keep the goal in sight. You may not need it forever, but for now, eat more omega

3's or take a supplement containing them everyday.

More information here at a recent study on BMC Complementary and Alternative Medicine www.biomedcentral.com/content/pdf/1472-6882-12-143.pdf[28]

This is just one of many studies demonstrating the positive effects of dietary fish oils & Omega 3's in reducing inflammation.

Calcium

Calcium is one of the most abundant minerals in our bodies. 99% of it is locked together with phosphorus and these compounds work together to make strong bones and hard teeth. Like everything in our body, these minerals move between blood and bones every day. Calcium is a muscle relaxer and plays a vital role in regulating our most important muscle, our heart. A balance of calcium is required for our heart muscle to relax and contract, and for the transmission of nerve impulses throughout the body. This is the same reason calcium helps as a natural anti-anxiety remedy. It's a natural muscle relaxer and prevents muscle cramps, including uterine cramps. [29-30]

The Recommended Daily Allowance (RDA) of calcium for women age 9-18 is 1,300 milligrams a day. The daily allowance decreases for women age

19-50 to 1,000 milligrams a day. Be aware that many of our foods come from calcium depleted soils and this makes it even more difficult to get the recommended daily allowance. A calcium supplement is easy to add to your daily diet. I prefer the liquid calcium. Always look for a calcium supplement that includes magnesium, vitamin D, omega-3 fatty acids and vitamin K (in particular K-2). Without these essential co-factors, the calcium may end up in our blood vessels rather than in our bones. A calcium "citrate" supplement is the most absorbable form of calcium.

Many brands of calcium can still be effective so find a brand you like and can afford. If you are still in the crucial bone building years, under age 22 then you should be participating in weight bearing exercise and taking a calcium supplement. Weight bearing exercises can be as easy as push ups and will be covered in more detail in the chapter on exercise. If you're taking "The Pill", adding calcium to your diet for just one year will reduce your risk of developing osteoporosis by 3-10%. Bones don't build up overnight. Like I've said before our bodies change gradually over time. We can't expect miracles in a day or two, but consistent effort will produce gratifying results.

Another option is to increase calcium rich foods. Bone broth soup, (slow cooking bones for days or even a week or more) is probably the best and cheapest way to get absorbable calcium. Just drink the water as soup broth or use the broth to make a soup or stem. This may take some effort, but remember this is part of long term changes that create better health throughout your entire life.

Try adding 3-4 calcium rich foods each day or supplement with a quality calcium supplement.

Calcium rich foods can be easy to add into your everyday diet. Below are a few of my favorite calcium rich foods and the milligrams of calcium they contain:

Almonds: 80 mg (1 ounce) A great on-the-go snack.
Sesame seeds: Sprinkle a handful on salads or a vegetable dish or add them to your trail mix.
Yogurt: 150-200 mg (1 cup) Try to eat organic milk products whenever possible.
Fish with bones in them, like sardines or canned salmon, are high in calcium. (ok not my favorite but very high in calcium)
Cottage cheese: 140 mg (1 cup) My favorite is with fresh pineapple.
Pinto Beans: 103 mg (1 cup) Love them in a burrito with fresh salsa!
Kale: 90 mg (1/2 cup) I like mine sautéed with onions and Himalayan salt.
Kidney Beans: 69 mg (1 cup) Add a few to a salad.

Black Beans: 46 mg (1 cup) A black bean burrito is quick to make and easy to take to the office for lunch.

Broccoli: 36 mg (1/2 cup) Steam lightly to protect all the good nutrients. Eating raw is a little hard for the digestive system.

Orange juice: Some orange juice is fortified with calcium and a little goes a long way. Don't make this a staple, but in moderation it will help your cause.

A final note on calcium:

Eating a diet high in protein can hinder calcium absorption. Osteoporosis, (soft bones, usually later in life) is now associated with excess protein intake as well as calcium insufficiency. The insufficiency is not necessarily due to a lack of calcium in our diets, but rather a lack of calcium *absorption*. This is why I recommend calcium rich foods over a calcium supplemental pill.

When we are overweight, the excess fat in our diets actually locks up calcium in the intestines... (another good reason to keep the fat off.) Vitamin D can help unlock some of the calcium needed for bone growth and stability. Consider a multi-vitamin that contains all the essential minerals for maximum health benefits. Also, remember to buy a calcium *citrate* supplement rather than calcium *carbonate*. The citrate variety is more absorbable.[31]

Preferably, look for a calcium supplement with a calcium/magnesium ratio of 1:1. This means equal amounts of calcium to magnesium. If the capsule contains 500 mg of calcium it should also contain 500 mg of magnesium. Sometimes this can be difficult to find, but there are many manufacturers who have changed their ratio because of new bone health research.

Magnesium Mg

Magnesium (Mg) doesn't seem to get enough press for all the hard work it does in the body. It's an essential mineral and a catalyst for many other functions. Without it our bodies CANNOT function optimally. Magnesium is essential for making new cells; it's needed to make bone and ATP- the body's fuel. Magnesium must be present for insulin secretion, heart function and healthy bowel function. Muscle cramps, blood clots and B vitamins all depend on magnesium to do their job. "Dietary intake of Mg in the U.S. is less than the recommended amount."[32] Some studies say 60-80% of the U.S. population is magnesium deficient. Ideally we should receive Mg through our food, however you can add 400 mg of magnesium daily in a supplement to help relieve menstrual cramps and increase healthy energy production.

In the past, our food provided enough of this trace mineral. Nuts and grains, beans, dark leafy vegetables such as kale, spinach, swiss chard, broccoli and pumpkin seeds are high in magnesium. Fish and some meats are also good sources for magnesium. Today, soil has been depleted of minerals and the amount of processed foods we eat does not supply what your body needs. This may sound repetitive but again, a quality multi- vitamin supplement will most likely be enough to replenish what you lack. You need a minimum of 300 mg of magnesium per day.

Magnesium has been studied extensively for cramps and uterine pain during menstruation.[34] Nutritional experts don't agree on whether equal amounts of magnesium and calcium should be supplemented, or a ratio of 2x as much calcium to magnesium. However, most experts agree that our magnesium deficiencies are extreme and most of us should supplement for a period of months to a year to stabilize our mineral balance. Magnesium is stored in and on our bones, and deficiencies often show up later in life. Create strong bones while you are young and maintain those bones as you age. This trace mineral is absolutely essential.

Why is this important?

Remember the "Play" in Chapter 2 and the role of Ester and Terone (progesterone)? The rise of progesterone after ovulation increases the body's storage of magnesium, zinc and vitamin B6. It also brings down the copper, which has gradually risen to a mid-cycle peak. If Terone fails to show up for his entire role, the body's necessary trace minerals also get thrown off.

Magnesium, zinc and B6 tend to be low and copper tends to rise causing a host of other problems. Mineral balance in our bodies is delicate and operates optimally when balanced within a very strict ratio. When our leading man cannot carry out his full performance, everyone else is also affected. The longer the imbalance continues the worse things can get.

Magnesium can be found in brown rice, spelt, quinoa, barley and rye. Spelt and quinoa are grains that can be found at most health food stores today and cooked like rice. You might be surprised how tasty they are!

TIP: As mentioned earlier, an Epson-Salt Bath is a great way to support a healthy mineral balance. Your skin will absorb the magnesium (and other minerals) your body needs by soaking for just 10-15 minutes in a hot bath. Start taking an epsom salt bath at least once a month. Right before your Period is a great time to pamper yourself with a 20 minute soak.

Zinc

Nearly 100 different enzymes depend on zinc for their ability to catalyze vital chemical reactions.[33] The reason it's an important supplement to add is because zinc is a multi-purpose trace mineral. Zinc is necessary for a woman's body to produce mature eggs at ovulation. It also helps maintain levels of estrogen, progesterone and testosterone and many other critical functions that occur every day. Zinc has become depleted in our soils and therefore lacking in our foods.

Generally a multivitamin will include 15 mg of zinc. If you are a strict vegetarian, zinc supplementation is critical. Your requirement for dietary zinc may be as much as 50% greater than the non-vegetarian because eating high amounts of grains and legumes produces higher levels of phytic acid which reduces zinc absorption. Zinc is sold as an individual supplement as well as it's inclusion in most multi-vitamin supplements.

Iodine

Iodine seems to be the most ignored trace mineral. Our thyroid gland cannot function without iodine and our bodies use this mineral for hundreds of functions every day.

Additionally there is lesser known, yet substantial research supporting iodine's role in balancing estrogen levels and supporting ovary health. Our ovaries hold a high concentration of iodine along with breast tissue. Most importantly, recent studies have shown iodine helpful for improving the metabolism of estrogen. For these reasons, iodine should not be overlooked as a supplement to your diet.

Iodine deficiency has been common for more than a generation in the mid-western region of the United States even after it was added to table salt. The World Health Organization (WHO) "estimated that over 30% of the world's population (2 billion people) have insufficient iodine intake" (Linus Paulings Institute-Oregon 2010). Research suggests iodine deficiency is a serious problem where diets are devoid of iodine containing foods such as seaweed and fish. Iodine was added to table salt years ago mainly to prevent goiters. Today table salt is often the only source of iodine for many of us.

You can have your iodine levels checked by a blood test. I recommend iodine drops daily for all my patients who show signs of estrogen dominance. For our purposes, supplementation at a very low dose is usually sufficient. Supplementing iodine in liquid form is easy and just 1-2 mg of iodine daily is both safe and effective. This is usually a few drops, check the bottle you purchase. You can put the drops right in your mouth or add to a little water. This is a simple and preventative way to be sure you are getting enough iodine every day.

Diindolylmethane - DIM

DIM has been getting more attention lately and can be found online and in most health food stores. As with all the supplements listed here, always check out the manufacturer and buy the highest quality you can find. I use DIM in my practice and find it quickly reduces breasts tenderness. Results vary depending on brands and dosage so consult with your health practitioner.

The following definition of diindolylmethane was taken from the *National Cancer Institute*:

DIM : A phytonutrient and plant indole found in cruciferous vegetables including broccoli, brussels sprouts, cabbage, cauliflower and kale, with potential antiandrogenic and antineoplastic activities. As a dimer of indole-3-carbinol, diindolylmethane (DIM) promotes beneficial estrogen metabolism in both sexes by reducing the levels of 16-hydroxy estrogen metabolites and increasing the formation of 2-hydroxy estrogen metabolites, resulting in increased antioxidant activity. Although this agent induces apoptosis in tumor cells in vitro, the exact mechanism by which DIM exhibits its antineoplastic activity in vivo is unknown. Check for active clinical trials using the

NCI Thesaurus. Some past studies here:
www.dimfaq.com/site/breasthealth.htm

DIM is another great addition to all the above supplements to speed up your body's transformation process and put you in the fast lane to ending the PMS & cramps.

Some of these supplements you may want to continue for months or years. Other supplements may only be needed until the majority of your symptoms have subsided and you have Stopped Your Bitching. Again, these are the minimum supplement requirements to help reduce Period pain. You may need others. Everyone is slightly different. I always advise everyone to try and get all these vitamins and minerals from foods first for your optimum health.

(Note: If you add up the cost of your montly supplements and spent some or all of that money on organic fruits and vegetables you would most likely not need the supplements.)

Your Part 7

This chapter also has a lot of information. You may want to read it more than once and then decide how much your health is worth! Regardless of what dollar figure you assign yourself, make it a realistic amount that you can spend on your health for the next six months to create real change. We'll call this the "HEALTHY ME" fund.

Remember, change doesn't happen overnight in our bodies.   Give yourself permission to spend this money and organize your budget so it is possible. This is the best investment you will ever make. Use this money on healthy foods, supplements and/or seeing a health care professional to help you along this journey Later you can decide how your "Healthy Me" will be used. **Right now, just make the promise to yourself**

My health is worth at least _____ per month.
I know making some health changes will cost a little money so I promise to commit for at least the next six months $ _____per month to improve my health. I will adjust my spending and save this money by making the following 5 changes. (Write these 5 changes and your promise down in the notebook you've been keeping or on the next page.

Sign_____Date_____

5 Changes I'm making to create and maintain a "Healthy Me'

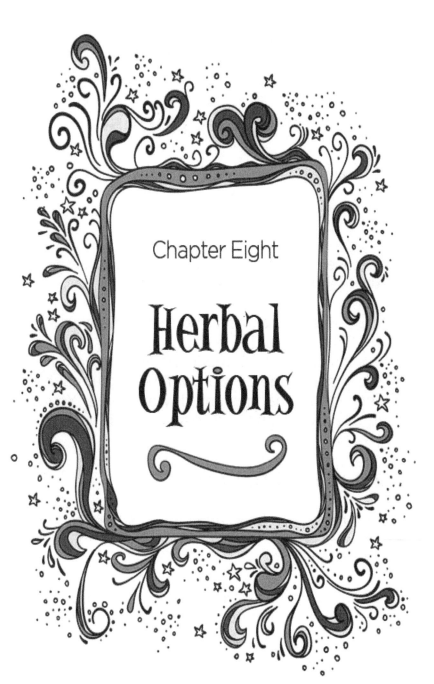

Chapter Eight

Herbal Options

Chapter 8

Herbal Options

YEAH! It's Day 8 and you're feeling great!

No excuse – no telling yourself this stuff is too hard. Keep Up all the good work.

Step by step you can do this.This is the way it is done. This is also the reason I wrote "30 Day's of Tips to: Stop Your Bitching...naturally" This companion guidebook. will help you make all the necessary changes one day at a time. You can even use it over and over every month to keep you on track.

NOW, Herbal Options

I know herbs can be confusing. It's hard to know which ones to trust and which ones you might be a waste of money.

I'm going to clear up this confusion for you. Just like all the other chapters, this one is packed full of information. A bit of background first on the herb/botanical world.

Three distinct types of herbal traditions are popular today: Traditional Chinese Medicine (TCM), Ayervedic Herbs and Western Herbalism. Each have their own history and although some of the same herbs/botanicals are shared by these three systems, many of the herbs are very different and used differently. I have expertise and training in all of these traditions, and for our purposes here I'm going to focus on those herbs that proved successful for my female patients who were dealing with PMS and menstraul irregularities.

Let's Start With the Oldest Medicine on Earth

Chinese Herbal Medicine has been practiced for thousands of years. If this book was published today for a Chinese, Taiwanese, Japanese or other Asian audience no explanation of the herbs below would be necessary. The herbs mentioned here are part of Asian culture and lifestyle. They are commonly found in corner drug stores and in food and drinks at the local convenient stores.

Some traditional pharmacies throughout Asia sell these herbs as roots, barks and berries. This is the raw form which needs to be taken home and boiled in water to drink as a tea. Other pharmacies sell only herbs in pills or herbs in small packets of powder which is much more convenient than having to boil your herbs.

In the United States, herbal tonics and formulas (especially Chinese herbs) are not our main healing modality and need some explanation. However, ginseng, a Chinese herb, is becoming popular in energy drinks which can now be found just about everywhere.

We Need A Reference Point

Let's use 1776, the year the United States of America was established for a reference point. This may help explain how long these herbs have been used.

China in 1776

In the year 1776, China had a well established government and a culture of mathematicians, scholars and doctors. The Great Wall of China had already been standing for some 1500 years. Chinese society depended upon its doctors for health just as we do today. The medicine and drugs that kept millions of people healthy had been in place for more than 1000 years, and is known today as Traditional Chinese Medicine (TCM) or Oriental Medicine, or Eastern medicine.

In 1776 there were over a thousand plants and minerals used in herbal medicine books. One of the most comprehensive herbal books on Chinese herbal medicine for women was written near the year 1776. The book covered the same topics on women's health we deal with today: Period pain, infertility, menopause, child birth recovery and more. The book became a standard for herbal formula combinations that worked for women's health. The herbal remedies written then are still used today. I think it's safe to say these herbal remedies are time-tested.

In China, the most complete herbal medicine book, the *Bencao Gangmu* was written over a period of nearly 30 years. It includes over 1800 drugs and Chinese herbs, 1100 illustrations and 11,000 herbal formula prescriptions for the treatment of 1094 diseases. It totals 52 volumes and is still published today in several languages. Chinese herbs have been used for over 2000 years. Today these same herbal combinations are covered by National Health insurance coverage in many Asian countries.

I'm providing this background because too often herbs are not considered a viable medical option. Yet, the very countries that invented much of our current technology for cell phones, T'V's and computers, have always used this system of medicine. I'm speaking of China, Taiwan and

Japan where herbs are included in their National Health Care system offered to all citizens.

Herbal formula combinations that were used for the last 2000 years have now been studied and validated by modern research and lab analysis. In fact, the same research has yielded many prescription drugs based on plant chemicals. Scientists know plants contain nutritional vitamins and substances such as flavonoids, tannins, polysaccharides and alkaloids which act like drugs in our bodies. Labs today can look at chemical markers in herbs with digital equipment and test for active constituents in plants.

Research has proven the many health benefits of botanical/herbal medicine. Clinical studies have been done on thousands of people and the results are measurable and remarkable. In many cases much more remarkable than drugs. Plant chemicals produce results that relieve our pain, help our moods and regulate our hormones. And of course all of these help us "Stop Our Bitching".

When combined, herbs can create particular healing effects. We call this a "synergy effect". It's a little like making a cake. If the flour, sugar, eggs and butter were all put into the oven in separate pans, you would not get a cake. But when these items are mixed together and cooked, we get a different result, we get a cake.

Herbal formulas often work the same way. In TCM, individual herbs mixed together in a combination with other herbs have enhanced effects. We know this from hundreds of years of practice, thousands and thousands of doctors writing thousands and thousands of formulas, using them on thousands and thousands of people for the last 2000 years.

A Study of The Studies

At the University of Western Sydney, in 2008, a large scale study was conducted on herbs used for menstrual irregularities. A team of world renowned researchers and scientists at the Cochrane Research Center reviewed this and other studies on herbal alternatives for primary dysmenorrhea (Period cramps). The Cochrane review "found promising evidence supporting the use of Chinese herbal medicine for primary dysmenorrhea". [36]

Their landmark decision came from studying 39 randomized controlled trials that together involved 3,475 women. Three trials compared Chinese herbal medicine with a placebo, one compared it with no treatment, two compared it with acupuncture, and one compared it with heat compression. They found the Chinese herbal remedies were significantly better at relieving painful cramps and other symptoms than acupuncture or a hot water bottle. [37]

The researchers gave women Chinese herbal formulas for their PMS and menstrual cramps. Herbs in the formulas included (but were not limited to) Chinese Angelica Root (Dang Gui), Nut-Grass Rhizome, Szechuan Lovage Root or Ligusticum, Red Peony Root, White Peony Root and Licorice Root.

So how do these herbs / botanicals work?

Most of the evidence on herbs shows that certain plants help to re-establish the normal balance of estrogen and progesterone during the menstrual cycle.(Remember Chapter 2) Below is a brief explanation of the ones from the research listed above that I have also found most effective in my practice.

Dang Gui – Dang Quai

Chinese Angelica Root -Dang Gui is considered an antispasmodic and has estrogen adaptogenic properties. This mean it adapts to what your body needs. Needs may vary between different women. Several new studies have examined and found that Dang Gui is an indispensable herb for PMS symptoms. Dang Gui is also considered the "women's ginseng" because of its plethora of well-established and proven actions. In Traditional Chinese Medicine (TCM), Dang Gui is rarely used alone and is typically used in combination with herbs such as peony (paeonia officinalis) for menstrual cramps.[38]

Dang Gui is considered a blood tonic herb which is warming and dispersing. The coumarin chemicals present in Dang Gui may help dilate blood vessels and relax the smooth muscles of the uterus, thus relieving menstrual cramps.

Nut Grass, Cyperus

This herb is commonly combined with Dang Gui for irregular menstruation and dysmenorrhea. Remember the "SYNERGY" effect I spoke about above? Just like a cake is better when a receipe of ingredients is followed in the right amounts. Some ingredients work better together. The same is true with herbs.

Nut Grass has a major role in regulating our liver energy and is known for its ability to help regulate our menstrual cycles and Period pain. Its actions are intensified when combined with other herbs such as Dang Gui and Bupleurum. The book, "The Grand Materia Medica" written approximately 200 AD states that Nut Grass is the "Commander-in-Chief of Qi (energy) disorders, and for gynecology, the Supreme Leader."[35] It is also called an "immortal herb for women" as far back as 1550 AD. Cyperus's known chemical constituents include volatile oils, flavonoids and proteins.

Peony Root

Red and white peony roots are considered liver tonics in Chinese medicine. By strengthening the liver, they help increase the efficiency of protein and fat metabolism, thus inhibiting the excessive synthesis of prostaglandins that may cause an over-active uterus and endometrial pain. Excessive prostaglandins have been implicated in menstrual irregularities. Peony root is known to nourish the liver, our main blood filter, and to regulate the menstrual cycle. In TCM, the liver and mentrual problems have an inter-connected relationship. When the liver is working optimally, menstrual blood is also in balance. The opposite is also true; therefore a Chinese medicine doctor will always consider the condition of the liver when faced with mentrual irregularities.

Ligusticum

This herb is known for its ability to improve blood circulation and promote the flow of "qi" or vital energy. "Blood stasis" is a common term in TCM and when this occurs there is usually a stagnation of energy in the liver channel. Symptoms such as moodiness, depression, irritability, menstrual cramps, backache and bloating are referred to as "Liver Qi Stagnation". Chinese medicinal herbs help repair the body's functions and move the Qi. This alleviates blood stasis and the pain associated with it. Herbs such as Ligusticum can also harmonize the liver energy and relieve the "Liver Qi Stagnation". When liver channel energy is moving smoothly, disharmonies such as PMS are reversed.

Licorice Root

Licorice is one of the few Chinese herbs that goes to all twelve channels of the body. Because it can enter all body channels, this herb is often used to guide other herbs into channels they could not otherwise effect. This is the beauty of Chinese Herbal Medicine;- the combining of herbs to develop new medicinal properties. Again, it's about the synergy.

Licorice helps with PMS and menstrual cramps because it moderates spasms and alleviates pain, especially in the abdomen and legs. The two major constituents of licorice are glycyrrhizin and flavonoids. Flavonoids are antioxidants known to improve circulation, relieve tissue damage and reduce inflammation. Other great sources of flavonoids include onion, garlic, basil, spinach and green leafy vegetables.

Where Do You Get These Herbs?

Thanks to modern science we know the herbs mentioned here work and are extremely safe. Herbal remedies can make PMS and cramps a thing of the past. These herbs are available in a product called PMS Relief Herb Pack by Pacific Herbs at www.pacherbs.com/.

I have prescribed PMS Relief Herb Pack for years. The combination of herbs in this product is very similar to TCM formulas written down hundreds of years ago.

I have found using PMS RELIEF HERB PACK for just a few days out of the month (during your Period and/or a day or two before your Period) can make a huge difference to end your pain and help resolve your PMS. PMS Relief Herb Pack can replace the NSAID's discussed in Chapter 4.

When you combine herbs with the other steps outlined in this book you will reach our goal, which is to "Stop Your Bitching...naturally".

Generally speaking you get more bang for your buck with a treatment protocol that includes plant based molecule because our bodies understand how to use these molecules. Our bodies have been using these molecules for thousands of years and studies have found less side effects associated with plant based molecules. I have found in my practice that using herbs is highly effective and without a doubt, reduces estrogen dominant symptoms, quickly..

Remember Chapter One... CHANGE?

In chapter one I spoke about the constant changes occurring in a woman's body throughout the month, similar to the endless cycles of the moon. The basis of TCM is change. It's called yin and yang. Now is your time to change! Don't put this off any longer. You deserve to be happy and you deserve a pain free life without Period cramps and PMS.

Popular Western Herbs

Herbs such as chasteberry, black cohosh, evening primrose oil, milk thistle and vitex are purported to relieve PMS symptoms in some women. Studies on these herbs reveal mixed results. Several studies found they were no more beneficial than a placebo. The National Institute of Health (NIH) did a systematic review in 2009 of many studies and their conclusion was "Only calcium had good quality evidence to support its use in PMS. Further research is needed, using RCTs of adequate length, sufficient sample size, well-characterized products and measuring the effect on severity of individual PMS symptoms." [39] However, many women have been using these Western herbs for years and see improvements with their use. I think if you find a high quality supplier and a high dose product, these herbs can help.

More on dose and packaging to follow. Often times it is not the herbs ineffectiveness but the lack of potency in the commercial product.

Black cohosh is approved in Germany for use in women with PMS. [40] This approval appears to be based on historical use rather than modern clinical trials. "Black cohosh may interact with many medications processed by the liver, including acetaminophen (Tylenol), atorvastatin (Lipitor), carbamazepine (Tegretol), isoniazid (INH),

methotrexate (Rheumatrex), and others." [41]
Research has suggested using Black cohosh for
more than 3-6 months has possible harmful effects
for the liver.

Milk thistle is an herb well known for its liver
detoxifying properties and can be very beneficial
for those with symptoms of estrogen dominance
(Look back at Chapter 3 for that symptom list).
Milk thistle also boosts glutathione levels which can
help eliminate poisons like heavy metals from the
body. In this way, Milk thistle protects the body
from oxidative stress.

Who's Herbal Products Should You Buy?

I use very specific practitioner lines of herbs in my
private practice. I hesitate to recommend specific
supplement manufacturers of herbs and vitamins
that do not meet the quality assurances of brands
available to health practitioners. I need to be
absolutely certain herbs are:
•Verified for proper herbal authenticity;
•Connected to a Certificate of Analysis (COA)
guaranteeing tested clean herbs, free from
pesticide residues
•Are packaged without unnecessary fillers and
additives.

If a supplement maker is unwilling to disclosure
where and by whom their products are
manufacturered, then you truly have no idea who

is making it and what is really inside. Who's watching the quality control? Often times it's the contract manufacturer. In that case, there is no guarantee onquality control and unfortuntately this is common place today in the supplement industry.

Purchase only premium trusted products from the most recognized and respected manufacturers. Anyone can contract to have dietary supplements made today and ingredients are commonly shipped from all parts of the globe. Don't be alarmed. Be aware that there is a lot of garbage on the market that has very little value. Companies that are not transparent about who or where their products are manufactured should not earn your trust.

On the other hand, there are some excellent manufacturers of supplements and herbs who operate under a gold standard. These companies have lot numbers and expiration dates on all their products. They don't use fillers and they perform a plethora of laboratory tests to satisfy strict guidelines before accepting an herbal ingredient or vitamin supplement into their warehouses. Only quality companies advertise their testing and processing. Many of the best supplement manufacturers provide this information on their websites. Another option, purchase your supplements and or herbs from a qualified health practitioner. They often have already done all this research.

Correct Dosing of Herbs

Herbs sold in pills and capsules often have such a small amount of herbs inside each capsule that they are ineffective unless a person uses about 20-30 capsules. Always check with a licensed practioner regarding the herbal products you take. It is very important *when researching an herb study to make sure you consider the dose of herbs used in the study and the dose you will be taking to get the same results.*

Currently, there are NO standardization requirements for herbal potencies and treatment protocols in the United States. Since herbs are natural substances, they DO degrade with time and temperature. Herbs exposed to high heat, light, air and moisture may not be as potent as when first dried or processed.

Unfortunately, it's nearly impossible in the U.S. to really know the potency of the product you are purchasing. This is why you must trust the manufacturer. Always look for the highest quality manufacturer and remember high quality products often times cost a bit more. The old saying you get what you pay for can be true in this case. Always do research on the dietary supplements you purchase.

Unlike many other countries, dietary supplements in the United States are not required to label the

percentage of excipients or fillers used in their products. Unfortunately, because herbs tend to clog up the machinery used to put them into pills or capsules, added filler may be as much as 50% of the product you receive.
 of the product you purchase. Yes, its shocking but true.

This is where professionals can be extremely important. You may want to discuss your herbal options with a Naturopathic Doctor, Acupuncturist, Chiropractor, Homeopathic Doctor, Oriental Medicine Doctor, or other licensed professional who has training in vitamins and herbal supplements. Many professionals sell brands of herbs and vitamins which are exclusive to medical professionals. Although many of these brands are a little more expensive, remember, "you get what you pay for".

Asking Your M.D. About Herbs

Medical doctors do not generally receive herbal training in school. In my experience, very few M.D.'s have any knowledge of herbal supplements or vitamin supplements. However, there is always an exception to the rule, and I encourage you to seek such an M.D. or a Complimentary and Alternative Medicine Practitioner (CAM) that has spent time learning about herbs and dietary supplements (vitamins). The more you learn here the more questions you might have. The next chapter will discuss CAM providers more thoroughly and how to find one near you.

One More Herbal Alternative

Mexican Yams are a plant within the yam family that are globally used to enhance woman's health. Yam roots contain saponins which naturally convert to progesterone. Research has shown that benefits from this root include PMS relief and reduction of hot flashes. This is just another example of allowing food to be thy medicine and medicine be thy food, as discussed earlier.

One Note About Natural Topical Progesterone

I often recommend progesterone topical creams for my patients. If you decide to use this type of cream you should start on the day you ovulate (or day before) and then continue for only 10-14 days. It is best **not** to use it everyday of the month. This will help mimic your body's natural cycle of hormones during the month. If you need to, refer back to Chapter 2 and look at the hormone chart.

For best results, combine progesterone cream with other steps discussed in previous chapters. Baby steps work but combining them moves you into the fast lane. You will get better results by combining the life style changes, the vitamins, herbs, the reduction of toxic chemicals and everything outlined in Chapter 6. These steps provide the momentum you need to sprint to the finish line. For more information or to purchase PMS Relief Herb Pack you can go to PacHerbs.com the Pacific Herbs website. www.pacherbs.com/

Your Part 8

Do some research on the dietary supplement products you already own. Grab the supplements in your kitchen or bathroom and do the research on them that I have mentioned above.

Check out who the manufacturer is and look them up on the Internet. Be a detective!

Learn as much as possible on your supplement manufacturers and do your own tests on various brands and see if you notice a difference in how you feel.

Consider purchasing high quality supplements from a licensed health provider trained in nutrition, vitamins and herbs.

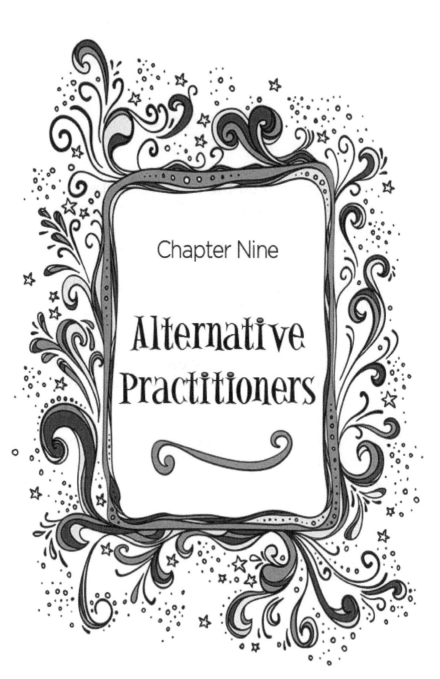

Chapter Nine

Alternative Practitioners

Chapter 9

Alternative Practitioners

Chiropractors, Acupuncturists, Homeopaths, Naturopathic Doctors and other Alternative Medicine healers all have treatments for menstrual cramps and PMS.

They can all help you Stop Your Bitching ...naturally! These professions all have stringent licensing requirements. In the U.S. these professionals complete a Bachelor's Degree (a 4 year degree) and then attend graduate school programs which often take 2-5 years to complete and have similar classroom requirements as med-school. Licensing requirements vary by state (Outside of the United States, please check for different requirements as they vary greatly).

Despite technological advances in Western medicine, health practitioners in "Complementary and Alternative Medicine" (CAM) can provide answers to many discomforts and diseases that Western medicine has difficulty treating.

What about the cost?Are they covered by my insurance?

It has become more common for Alternative Medicine Practitioners to be covered by your insurance plan. Call your provider and ask, you may be surprised. If you find a practitioner that you click with, talk to them about payment options. Many will be flexible with their fees and accept insurance payments even though they often don't cover the true cost of their services. Many will also work out payment plans. Remember your health is everything in life. If you don't have your health what do you have? Make your wellness a top priority.

What You Might Learn from A CAM Practitioner

This is an example of information you might hear from an Alternative Practitioner. I often teach my patients many ways to be in touch with their bodies.

Body Clues:

There are many clues your body gives you about your menstrual cycle each month. When you understand these clues it's reassuring that you are in tune with your bodies functions. The Play in Chapter 2 gave you the basic hormone ups and downs, but there is another way to know when you're ovulating and when to expect your Period. Cervical mucus holds lots of these clues. You can recognize your body's natural rhythms like ovulation by understanding the changes in cervical mucus. It's easy!

You know what mucus looks like when you blow your nose. Well, cervical mucus is similar in some respects. You can't blow it out but you can check your underwear. The word cervix is Latin for "the neck of the womb". In English, it is the top part of the vagina.

Throughout the month small amounts of mucus are discharged. This is perfectly normal and a good sign that your body is healthy. Cervical mucus has a few purposes, but mostly it is created to nourish and provides a safe environment for sperm.

All you have to do is check the mucus in your underwear (excreted from your vagina) whenever you go the bathroom. It's no big deal so don't get grossed out. Nobody else is going to know you're doing this either, so don't worry. It's your right and responsibility.

If you start becoming a detective and charting your cervical mucus you will be surprised how easy it is to know when you are ovulating. Below is an easy explanation on the changes which occur each month. Once you learn the pattern, and follow the changes throughout a month you will find it easier to predict when you are ovulating. Ovulation should be a half way point in your monthly cycle and with this information you can predict what hormones are affecting your mood and what to expect next.

For a woman with a 28-32 day cycle, the pattern of changes in her cervical mucus will look like this.

- **Days 1-5**: Menstruation – bleeding. No mucus.
- **Days 6-9**: Vagina is dry with little to no mucus.
- **Days 10-12**: Sticky, thick mucus appears, gradually becoming less thick and more white.
- **Days 13-15**: Mucus becomes thin, slippery, stretchy, and clear, similar to the consistency of egg whites. This is the most fertile stage.
- **Days 16-21**: Mucus becomes sticky and thick again.
- **Days 22-28**: Vagina becomes dry.

If your cycle is a little longer or shorter don't worry. Adjustments within a few days are perfectly normal.

Now predicting and knowing when you are ovulating is a piece of cake. Knowing why you're moody or irritable is now more understandable and with this information you can choose more rational decisions rather than emotionally charged ones.

Other Tips You Might Hear In My Office

In Western medicine we don't think about our uterus catching a cold, but often the diagnosis of a "cold uterus" alone can be the main reason you have excruciating menstrual cramps and this can affect fertility as women age. Keep in mind this is not the only reason, but it's a good place to start.

Chinese medicine relates some cramping and pain to a stagnation of blood and when the uterus is cold the blood congeals and causes pain. This is often why many women will use a heating pad or hot bath for cramp relief. Although this may sound too simple to believe, it really is that easy. Remember, this may not be the only reason for your cramps and pain. The body is a complex machine.

If a heating pad helps your Period cramps, you probably have a little too much cold, and not enough heat in the lower abdomen. There are fairly simple things you can do to prevent "a cold uterus".

Avoid simple activities like consuming an excess of cold beverages, sitting on cold snow, ice or concrete for any length of time, swimming in cold water on a regular basis and during menstruation, getting soaked in cold rain or wading through cold water. These are a few of the external causes which can cause cold within the body.

Internal cold and "Cold Uterus" can be caused by eating too many cold or raw foods. Internal cold may also occur after an illness or surgery when we are in a weakened state. Simple prevention techniques and awareness is all that is necessary to reduce internal cold including "cold uterus syndrome".

 If you are not getting enough answers from your MD, look for an Alternative Health Practitioner in your community. The links below will help you find practitioners near you.

Links to Find CAM Practitioners

(Complementary & Alternative Medicine)

For Acupuncturists look here:
www.tryacupuncture.org/

For Chiropractors look here:
www.findachiropractor.com/

For Homeopathic Physicians check here:
www.homeopathicdirectory.com/

For Naturopathic Doctors look here:
www.naturopathic.org/

For MD's who practice holistic and alternative medicine check here: www.womeninbalance.org/

Schedule consultations to talk with any of these professionals about how they can help you. You have nothing to lose and everything to gain. Consultations are usually free but not always so definitely ask. Many times a phone conversation may be enough to tell whether you're a good fit with a practitioner. If a particular professional does charge for consultations, simply ask the receptionist for 10 minutes of their time, a meet and greet basically. I've never had any doctor charge for 10 minutes and you'll get a quick impression if this is someone you want to work with. Often that's all it takes.

Self Massage and Acupressure

There are some things you don't need a health professional to do, and I'm going to teach you two places on your body that you can use your own two hands to help the physical symptoms that come with your "Period" pain.

In Traditional Chinese Medicine, the points I'm going to teach you here are referred to as Spleen 6 and Spleen 10, or Three Yin Intersection and Sea of Blood.

These two points are often used in an Acupuncture treatment to resolve stagnation of blood and energy in the liver, spleen and kidney channels. Acupuncture is all about bringing balance back to into your body. There are so many studies on acupuncture for pain relief I can't possibly mention them all here.

All you really need to remember is:

Stagnation = Imbalances = PAIN

Self massage or pressure on these points will help relieve stagnation and reduce pain during your menstrual cycle. You can use these points on any day of the month, but they are especially helpful right before your Period starts.

You'll want to massage these specific points for at least five (5) minutes each morning and night to reduce the stagnation in your liver, spleen and kidney channels. These channels affect what's going on in your uterus, also called the Mansion of Blood in Chinese medicine. Great translation, right? Sometimes it really feels like a "Mansion of Blood".

Five minutes may seem like a long time, but it's really not and your mansion of blood (uterus) will really thank you. Don't be afraid to do it more often, sitting at a desk, in a class or meeting. Sometimes nobody will know but you, so go for it. Anytime it feels good is fine.

Here is where you will find these very special points.

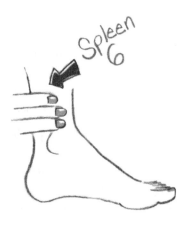

Spleen 6 or Three Yin Crossing is on the inside side of your leg just 3 fingers above your ankle bone that protrudes. The large bony protrusion is called the medial maleolus. You will know spleen 6 because it will feel tender when pushed firmly and when you slide your fingers just off the your leg bone, the tibia. Make sure you are on the inside (medial) part of your leg... big toe side is the medial side.

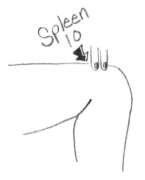

Spleen 10 – you can easily find this point when your knee is bent. The point is two finger above your knee cap, (patella) on the bulge of your thigh muscle (quadriceps femoris). An easy way to find this point is to take your right hand and place it on your right knee cap. The point is generally where your thumb rests.

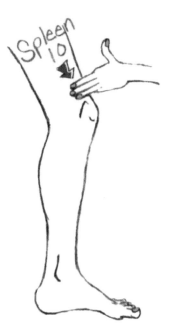

Push firmly into the point with your finger or knuckle and move in a circular motion to massage it thoroughly. It doesn't really matter if you do your left side or your right. Try both sides for both points and see which is most tender. Tender spots are a good place for you to massage.

Please note. Spleen 6, Three Yin Crossing is never used on pregnant women because it is so effective at moving blood.

Your Part 9

If you are not getting enough answers from your MD, look for an Alternative Health Practitioner in your community.

LOOK ONLINE FOR REVEIWS OF PRACTITIONERS NEAR YOU.
I have also provided links of where you can find them.

Schedule consultations. If a particular professional charges for consultations simply ask the receptionists for 10 minutes of their time...for a meet and greet.

If you don't feel you need additional medical advice beyond your MD right now, then your job is to read more about each of these modalities on the internet and see what they have to offer. You may change your mind once you know a bit more about CAM practitioners.

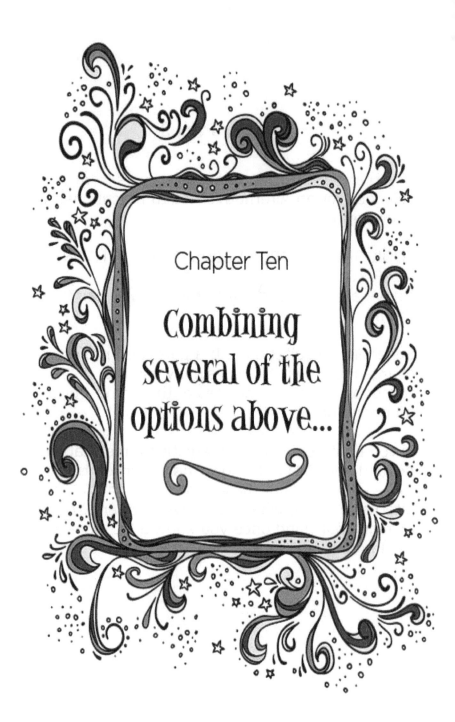

Chapter Ten

Combining several of the options above...

Chapter 10

Combining Several Of The Options Above

Hopefully you followed the instructions and you are now on the tenth day of reading a chapter a day. If you read the whole book in one day then please go back to the chapters that have boatloads of information (like Chapter 6) and give yourself some time with all the ideas and lifestyle changes presented there.

Today is Day 10! Hopefully you have learned a lot of new things in the last nine days. All this new information and life style changes are going to take some time to implement. Don't expect to do everything outlined all at once. You need to add little changes everyday, not all at once.

To help you through the first 31 days of changes, I've written a Guidebook to help you day by day This is an easy and fun way to start implementing all the action steps in this book. It help you get the most bang for your buck by doing certain changes on key days of your cycle. It also helps you maintain the new mindset around the way you approach your menstrual cycle.

You can always go back and re-read sections, but now it is time to bring all this information together to create a lasting change in your body and your health.

It's time to decide what steps you will take. The work is all outlined for you. To guide you along you may want to get "*30 Days of Tips to* Stop Your Bitching...naturally!" The companion guide to this book.

Remember Chapter 1 only a short 9 days ago? You read about attitude change. Go back there and look at this again. I hope you've been doing the 1 minute visualizations every night before bed and first thing in the morning. See yourself healthy, happy and energized. See yourself having fun and doing the things you love during your period.

This type of visualization is part of an inner dialogue that will become easier and easier as you practice it. This inner dialogue with your consciousness can and will become your outer reality. Get rid of thoughts that are self-defeating and unhappy, i.e. (I can't do this, it's too hard), or fearful thoughts, (I'm scared to try something new like acupuncture etc.). These are all self-limiting beliefs. These types of thoughts serve no good purpose!

They are self-sabotaging and self-loathing thoughts. If said to another person, these thoughts would be hurtful and damaging. How many times a day do you think, "I'm too fat, I'm not pretty, I'm not smart"? This is just plain RUDE!

Why do you say this to yourself?
There is no reason to tell yourself rude, hurtful stories like "you aren't good enough. . . blahh blahh blahhhh!". Change your attitude right now!

There is no "I can't do this". There is, however, "I don't want to do this!". Okay, if you don't want to make these changes then nobody can force you so stop reading right now. If you choose not to do anything about your body then that is your right, and your choice!

Remember Dr. Seuss

You have brains in your head. You have feet in your shoes. You can steer yourself any direction you choose!

(I love Dr. Seuss because he alwaysmade sense in such simple ways.)

Choose to steer yourself on a new healthy road. If the road today is pain free Periods, then you now have <u>everything</u> you need to get there. All you have to do is commit to stay on this road for at least 30 days and begin the lifestyle changes that are necessary and outlined in the chapters above.

Truth is, all you really need to do is love yourself, because it is the one relationship you are in for life. When you love yourself, you will want to give yourself the best body and the best health possible.

Love yourself because it's a very personal relationship.

It's forever, and the more you love yourself, the more you will be able to spread that love out to others.

When you feel good, those around you can feel good. Another way of saying this is: When you "Stop Your Bitching", life is not only easier for you, but for those around you.
So no more poking yourself all day with thoughts like "my body will never be that healthy"... because if you think that then I guarantee it will also become your reality.

On the other hand, if your thoughts are...

"I am beautiful and I treat my body with healthy food and healthy activities every day".

"I am always building new healthy cells in my body every day. My old outdated unhealthy cells are being replaced with the new and improved healthy cells every minute of every day."

"I am a beautiful girl, (woman, daughter mother, sister),_____(fill in the blank) and I deserve to be happy."

These thoughts will help you create a harmonious and loving relationship with yourself.

Treating yourself with self-respect and love on the inside is the first step to healing everything on the outside. Make your mind your best friend.

You started this new way of thinking in Chapter 1. Now you're graduating from more than just a one minute nightly visualization to really changing your every thought.

Start on the action steps that you wrote down in the "Your Part" at the end of each chapter.
One by one, take each chapter and make one or two changes every day.

Have you reduced the toxic load of endocrine disrupting chemicals that you put on your body under the disguise of "personal care products"?

Are you changing your diet? Are you trying some herbs and other supplements?

Have you joined an exercise class with a friend who will exercise with you?

Are you cutting down the junk food and eliminating HFCS?

Did you get your paraben-free water bottle?

Now is your decision time.

You cannot change your genetics, but you can change your health. You can control what you eat, how much you exercise and what you think about.

You can improve the health of your body with thousands of little decisions you make every day. I believe in prevention over treatment. Food should be your first medicine, so always begin by looking closely at what you eat and drink.

Begin today, it is never too late to change your body, change your moods and change your health.

You begin where you are. Wherever your starting point is doesn't matter.

You will notice a difference in the first month and these changes will begin to motivate you to stay on the path to improve your long term health.

Put an end to your menstrual cramps. Your days in bed and on the couch can become a foggy memory. The mood swings, depression and irritability no longer rule your life.

You can be in control of the way your body operates. You can control your natural hormone fluctuations with the foods you eat, the supplements you take, the exercise you get and the choices you make daily.
Emotional and physical wellness is a path that you must choose. It doesn't happen magically, it happens because you create it.

Create it first in your thoughts and then in your everyday actions.

Your Part 10

Now you should be ready to get started with all the information you learned here. I've made it easy to do this with:

<u>30 Day's of Tips To Stop Your Bitching...naturally!</u>

This companion guide has 31 helpful hints to keep you on the right path the first month and every month thereafter. You can use it over and over again. Printed as a notebook for you to keep your own notes on your progress, day by day.

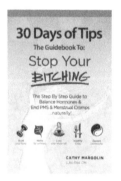

You can find this book on Amazon & other online stores or the Pacific Herbs website.www.PacHerbs.com

This book makes it fun and easy to stay on track and put all this new information to work for you... everyday.

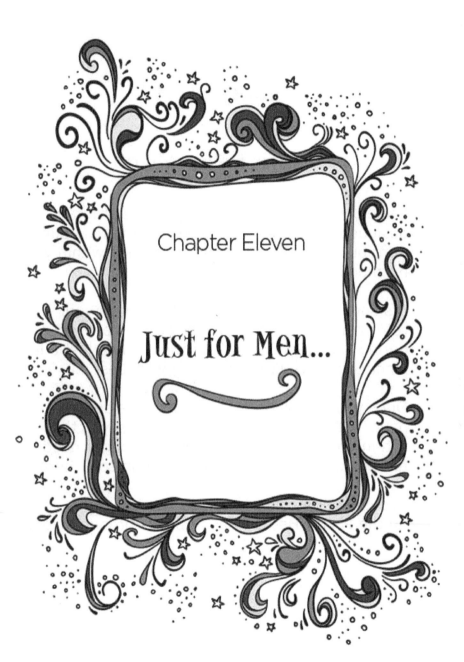

Chapter Eleven

Just for Men...

Chapter 11

Just For Men

Ladies, while you are working on the program designed here I have a gift for the men in your life. Print out this little chart for every man within your hormonal reach.

It's something you may want to post on your refrigerator, bathroom mirror or even at work during your "Period" to help the men be just a little kinder when you're not feeling your best.

Once you complete the program here and you have "Stopped Your Bitching...naturally!", those within your hormonal reach will no longer need this fun and crazy chart. Sorry it's not in color here.

You can get a color download version of this chartg on the Pacific Herbs website books product page.

<u>Survival Tips For Men:</u>
How To Talk To A Woman
While She's PMS'ing

Dangerous	Safer	Safest	Super Safe
What's for dinner?	Can I help you with dinner?	I'll go get some take out.	Here, have some chocolate
Are you wearing that?	I've always loved you in those sweatpants.	Wow! Look at You!	Here, have some chocolate
What are you so worked up about?	Maybe we're overreacting?	Here take my wallet.	Here, have some chocolate
Should you be eating that?	You know, there are a lot of apples left.	Can I get you a glass of wine with that?	Here, have some chocolate
What did YOU do all day?	I hope you didn't over-do-it today.	You had a hard day do you want a massage?	Here, have some chocolate
Are you having cramps today?	I know exactly how you feel.	Let me get you a bottle of painkillers.	Here, have some chocolate

Review This Book

One last thing...if you bought this book on Amazon, they give you the opportunity to rate this book. Please take a moment to do this! F this book has helped you please tell other woman too. Or share your on your Facebook, Twitter. Or other social sites. If you believe this book is worth sharing, please take a few seconds to let your friends know about it!

If it makes a difference in their life, they will be forever grateful to you.

Be Well,
Cathy

Suggestions for food choices:

Below is a laundry list of healthy food choices. Read through
them and decide which ones you can enjoy eating immediately.
Then choose one new food a day and start changing your body
from the inside out!!

Your body is a temple and you need to treat it like one.

The goal here is to eat a healthy nutrient-dense diet that
reduces the excess amount of estrogen in your body. This will
help balance your natural hormone levels along with reducing
menstrual irregularities and mood swings.

Your meat must be HORMONE FREE!! There is SO much
crap in our meat these days it's really disgusting. Injecting
animals with hormones is not the path to a better burger. Add
to that the horrific treatment of the animals and I can hardly
look a chicken or cow in the face. It is your choice to eat meat
or not but when you do, consciously choose to eat it without
hormones. If you can't afford organic, hormone free meat try a
vegetarian burger or add tempeh to your meal instead of
chicken. There are enough recipe books, websites and cooking
shows to help you with this one.

No soy!! You read it correctly.   NO SOY!   That includes
products that say "LECITHIN" .... This is just another name for
soy. Today's soy is 90% genetically modified (GMO). GMO's
are unsafe and untested in humans. Soy also boosts your
estrogen production. If you read Chapter 3 on estrogen
dominance you understand why you need to reduce your
estrogen, not increase it right now. Soy/lecithin is in nearly
every processed food so read the labels carefully and when you
see lecithin, put it back on the shelf.

Don't get me wrong, there are benefits to organic soy foods and I usually highly recommend fermented soy foods such as tempeh and miso. However, the chemical structure of soy is very similar to the chemical structure of human estrogen. This is why it is often referred to as a plant estrogen or phyto-estrogen. When your PMS and cramps are under control, you have regular menstrual cycles and you have no estrogen dominance symptoms, then, and only then can you add organic soy into your diet. Right now, while we are eliminating excess estrogen (which is usually more than abundant during our younger reproductive years), there is no reason to add it to your diet.

Cut back on wheat. Gluten free breads and pasta are easy to find. Brown rice and quinoa are really tasty and a great option instead of wheat. Faro is a grain, high in protein and a fantastic replacement for rice.

Easy on the tomatoes

Tomatoes are highly acidic, and can irritate your system. The endometriosis causes your body to be inflamed internally, so cutting back is essential. Additionally, if you are eating canned tomatoes, or tomato sauce coming from a can you are also eating BPA's. Remember BPA's are chemicals that should not be in our foods. Canning manufacturers use this chemical and canned tomatoes are particularly bad because their acid breaks down the BPA lining of the cans and end up in our food. Stop eating those fast-food pizzas and make your own with a glass jar of tomato sauce. If you love tomatoes and grow them at home then go ahead, a few won't hurt.

No dairy except a little scoop of non-fat organic yogurt on meals if you like. For a milk substitute, use almond milk or rice milk which comes in a variety of flavors. Soy milk is really fattening, has phyto-estrogens your body does not need and many soy milk products are genetically modified (GMO) soy. If you must drink soy milk make sure to buy organic soy. If you absolutely insist on having cow's milk in your diet make sure it is rBGH FREE, that means HORMONE FREE.   It absolutely needs to say ORGANIC or RAW!! If it does not contain these words do not drink it.

Say Yes to organic! No genetically modified foods. Try to buy organic fruits and vegetables whenever possible but at the very least WASH all your fruits and vegetables with a good natural produce cleanser, or soak in the sink with the soap for a while to get the wax or any dirt and chemicals off. It's the CHEMICALS that you want to avoid.

NO ALCOHOL. Consider substituting Kombucha (a drink with probiotics and enzymes) for alcohol. Kombucha drinks can be found at most health food stores and comes in a great array of flavors. It is delicious and sooo healthy. No alcohol may be difficult to wrap your mind around (if you are of legal age to drink) but consider that all alcohol is processed in your liver. Right now your liver does not need more work to do.

Very little to No sushi This might be torture for some of you but there are a LOT of unwanted pollutants in raw fish today. If you love fish, go ahead and eat it cooked. Know where the fish was caught and try to buy non-farm raised whenever possible.

Cut the Crap. Artificial sweeteners make a mess of your endocrine system. **Sugar** is almost just as bad. To really curb your sugar habit, try the honey trick discussed earlier. Start cutting back where you can but don't make yourself crazy over this one.   Sugar is addictive and this is hard for everyone.

Cooked food not raw! Raw food is harder to digest. Cooking foods helps release enzymes which make it easier to digest.

Grains: Sweet rice, brown rice, black rice, millet, pearl barley, oats.

Vegetables: Onion, yellow & green scallion, squash, winter squash, sweet potatoes, turnip, green chili peppers, eggplant, caper, anise, kohlrabi, leek, garlic, fresh mustard leaf.

Organic Meat: Chicken, beef, lamb, leg of lamb, animal livers (chicken beef, lamb), turkey.

Shellfish: Sea cucumber, shrimp, lobster.

Fish: Anchovy, Butterfish, Catfish, Common carp, Sardine (fresh), Salmon, Mussel, Shrimp/Prawn, Trout.

Fruits & nuts: Chestnut, peanut, sunflower seeds, walnut, coconut milk, pine kernel, walnut, strawberry, cherry, dates, black orange, peach, longan, lychee, papaya.

Dairy: Real Butter

Oils: Peanut oil, walnut oil, sunflower oil, blended oils.

Spices: Pepper (black), rosemary, savory, basil, bay, cayenne, chili, chive seed, cardamom seed, cinnamon bark, clove, coriander seed, dill seed, fennel seed, ginger (dry), jasmine, ginger (fresh), juniper, nutmeg.

Other foods: Malt sugar (better than cane sugar), vinegar.

Just a Fun Fact: Women who live together often get their periods around the same time. There are a few reason women's cycles tend to synchronize, moon cycles may be one and another has to do with odorless chemicals called "pheromones" (sounds like hormones). Pheromones are detected by our bodies and respond to the pheromones of women around us. Gradually this creates a synchronicity of menstrual cycles. If you live with one or more menstruating women, you'll probably notice you get your cycles at the same time each month or within a few days of each other.

REFERENCES

Chapter 2

1. Medscape Medical News President's Cancer Panel: Environmental Cancer Risk Underestimated

2.http://www.medscape.com/viewarticle/721766?sssdmh=dm1.616851&src=nldne&uac=139834FJ

Chapter 3

3 High-throughput screening and mechanism-based evaluation of estrogenic botanical extracts Cassia R. Overka, Ping Yaoa, Shaonong Chena, Shixing Dengb, Ayano Imaia, Matthew

Maina, Andreas Schinkovitza, Norman R. Farnswortha, Guido F. Paulia, and Judy L. Boltona, A UIC/NIH Center for Botanical Dietary Supplements Research & Pharmacognosy, College of Pharmacy, University of Illinois at Chicago, Chicago, IL 60612

Chapter 4

Herbs treat acetaminophen liver damage.
UCLA - Univ. of California Los Angeles: "Caution advised when using Acetaminophen"
http://www.nlm.nih.gov/medlineplus/druginfo/meds/a681004.html

The structural basis for the prevention of nonsteroidal antiinflammatory drug-induced gastrointestinal tract damage by the C-lobe of bovine colostrum lactoferrin. Mir R, Singh N, Vikram G, Kumar RP, Sinha M, Bhushan A, Kaur P, Srinivasan A, Sharma S, Singh TP.Department of Biophysics, All India Institute of Medical Sciences, New Delhi, India.
http://www.ncbi.nlm.nih.gov/pubmed/20006955

Over the counter non-steroidal anti-inflammatory drugs and risk of gastrointenstinal bleeding **Authors:** Blot W.[1]; Mclaughlin J.[1] **Source:** Journal of Epidemiology and Biostatistics, Volume 5, Number 2, 1 February 2000 , pp. 137-142(6) **Publisher:** Martin Dunitz Ltd, part of the Taylor & Francis Group

J; Henry, D (March 2000). "Consumption of NSAIDs and the development of congestive heart failure in elderly patients: an underrecognized public health problem" (Free full text). *Archives of internal medicine* 160 (6): 777–84. doi:10.1001/archinte.160.6.777. ISSN 0003-9926. PMID 10737277. http://archinte.amaassn.org/cgi/pmidlookup?view=long&pmid=10737277.ht tp://www.ncbi.nlm.nih.gov/pubmed/19568687

http://www.bmj.com/cgi/content/full/332/7553/1302?view=long&pmid=167
40558

http://archinte.ama-assn.org/cgi/content/full/160/6/777

Moore, De (2002). "Drug-induced cutaneous photosensitivity: incidence, mechanism, prevention and management". *Drug safety : an international journal of medical toxicology and drug experience* 25 (5): 345–72. doi:10.2165/00002018-200225050-00004. ISSN 0114-5916. PMID 12020173.

Chapter 5

12. Cochrane Database Syst Rev. 2001;(4):CD002120. *Combined oral contraceptive pill (OCP) as treatment for primary dysmenorrhea. Proctor ML, Roberts H, Farquhar CM. Department of Obstetrics and Gynecology, National Women's Hospital, Claude Road, Epsom, Auckland, New Zealand, 1003. m.proctor@auckland.ac.nz Update in: Cochrane Database Syst Rev. 2009;(2):CD002120. http://www.ncbi.nlm.nih.gov/pubmed/11687142*

13. Panzer C, Wise S, Fantini G, Kang D, Munarriz R, Guay A, and Goldstein I. Impact of oral contraceptives on sex hormone-binding globulin and androgen levels: a retrospective study in women with sexual dysfunction. J Sex Med 2006;3:104–113.

14. Schiefer HG (1997). "Mycoses of the urogenital tract". Mycoses 40 Suppl 2: 33–6. PMID 9476502.

15. Geburtshilfe Frauenheilkd. 1981 Sep;41(9):630-4.New results in connection with the problem of a connection between oral contraception and vaginal yeast 5541 http://www.ncbi.nlm.nih.gov/pubmed/6922063

16. Indian J Nutr Diet. 1984 Jul;21(7):225-32. Effect of oral contraceptives on the nutrient profile of women belonging to high income group http://www.ncbi.nlm.nih.gov/pubmed/12268340

17. Nutritional effects of oral contraceptive use: a review. Journal of Reprodictive Medicine. 1980 Oct;25(4):150-6. http://www.ncbi.nlm.nih.gov/pubmed/7001015

18. Linus Pauling Institute, Micronutrient Research for Optimum Health Oregon

19. Linus Pauling Institute, Micronutrient Research for Optimum Health Oregon http://lpi.oregonstate.edu/infocenter/vitamins/vitaminC/

20. www.mayoclinic.com

21. http://www2.cochrane.org/reviews/en/ab004425.html

22.http://jcem.endojournals.org/cgi/content/full/90/9/5127?maxtoshow=&H
ITS=10&hits=10&RESULTFORMAT=1&title=oral+contraceptives&andorexactt
itle=and&andorexacttitleabs=and&andorexactfulltext=and&searchid=1&FIRSTINDEX=0&sortsp
ec=relevance&resourcetype=HWCIT

23. Journal of Adolescence Health. 2004 Dec;35(6):427-9. Depot
medroxyprogesterone acetate, oral contraceptives and bone mineral density
in a cohort of adolescent girls.
http://www.ncbi.nlm.nih.gov/pubmed/15581522
Low-dose oral contraceptive use significantly increases the risk of both
cardiac and vascular arterial events events.Pubmed Data : J Clin Endocrinol
Metab. 2005 Jul;90(7):3863-70. Epub 2005 Apr 6. PMID: 15814774 Jul 01,
2005
Oral contraceptive use increases the risk for premenopausal breast cancer. P
ubmed Data : Mayo Clin Proc. 2006 Oct;81(10):1290-302. PMID: 17036554
Oct 01, 2006 Study Type : Meta Analysis
Six studies in the medical literature have demonstrated an increased risk for
liver cancer between 2- and 20- fold in longer durations of oral contraceptive
use. Pubmed Data : J Hepatol. 2007 Oct;47(4):506-13. Epub 2007 Apr 5.
PMID: 17462781

The risk of ischemic stroke is increased in current oral contraceptive
users.Pubmed Data : JAMA. 2000 Jul 5;284(1):72-8. PMID: 10872016 Jul
05, 2000Study Type : Meta Analysis

There is an increased risk for inflammatory bowel disease in oral
contraceptive agent users. Pubmed Data : Gut. 1995 Nov;37(5):668-73.
PMID: 8549943   Nov 01, 1995 Study Type : Meta Analysis

Among women over age 35 years at diagnosis, compared with never users,
those who had used oral contraceptives for 3 or more years during the past
5 years were at a 2.54-fold increased risk of breast cancer. Pubmed. Breast
Cancer Res Treat. 1998 Jul;50(2):175-84. PMID: 9822222 Jul 01, 1998

Levonorgestrel and ethinylestradiol oral contraceptive use results in lower
levels of total and free testosterone in women.   Pubmed Data :
Contraception. 1994 Dec;50(6):563-79. PMID: 7705098 Dec 01, 1994

Long-term oral contraceptive use among young women or use beginning
near menarche may be associated with a small excess breast cancer risk.
Natl Cancer Inst. 1994 Apr 6;86(7):505-14. PMID: 8133534   Apr 06, 1994

Low dose combined oral contraceptives result in wide fluctuations in
hemostatic markers in women. Clin Appl Thromb Hemost. 1999 Jan;5(1):60-
70. PMID: 10725985   Jan 01, 1999

Oral contraceptive agents are associated with an increased risk for the development of irritable bowel disease. Am J Gastroenterol. 2008 Sep;103(9):2394-400. Epub 2008 Aug 5. PMID: 18684177 Sep 01, 2008

Oral contraceptive use is associated with increased breast cancer risk and increased malignancy among young women. J Natl Cancer Inst. 1995 Jun 7;87(11):827-35. PMID: 7791232 Jun 07, 1995

Oral contraceptive use>or =1 year was associated with a 2.5-fold increased risk for triple-negative breast cancer. Cancer Epidemiol Biomarkers Prev. 2009 Apr;18(4):1157-66. Epub 2009 Mar 31. PMID: 19336554 Apr 01, 2009

Parabens detection in different zones of the human breast: consideration of source and implications of findings. J Appl Toxicol. 2012 May;32(5):305-9. doi: 10.1002/jat.2743. Epub 2012 Mar 7. Harvey PW, Everett DJ.http://www.ncbi.nlm.nih.gov/pubmed/22408000

Chapter 6

**Best book on food temperatures & Chinese Nutrition is "
The Tao of Nutrition by Maoshing Ni & Cathy McNease.**

24. Center for Disease Control Prevention National Report on Human Exposure to Environmental Chemicals Fact Sheet Bisphenol A (BPA) http://www.cdc.gov/exposurereport/BisphenolA_FactSheet.html

25. American Cancer Society
http://www.cancer.org/docroot/MBC/content/MBC_2_3x_Exercise.asp?sitearea=MBC

Urinary bisphenol A concentrations and their implications for human exposure in several Asian countries
Pubmed Data : Environ Sci Technol. 2011 Aug 15 ;45(16):7044-50. Epub 2011 Jul 20. PMID: 21732633
Article Published Date : Aug 15, 2011
Study Type : Human Study
Diseases : Bisphenol-A Toxicity : CK(46) : AC(10)

Bisphenol A acts as an endocrine disruptor in relation to serum thyroid and reproductive hormone levels in men from an infertility clinic.
Pubmed Data : Environ Sci Technol. 2010 Feb 15;44(4):1458-63. PMID: 20030380
Article Published Date : Feb 15, 2010
Study Type : Human Study
Diseases : Bisphenol-A Toxicity : CK(46) : AC(10), Infertility: Male : CK(209) : AC(52), Low Testosterone : CK(385) : AC(70)

BPA is positively associated with generalized obesity, abdominal obesity, and insulin resistance in middle-aged and elderly Chinese adults.
Pubmed Data : J Clin Endocrinol Metab. 2011 Nov 16. Epub 2011 Nov 16. PMID: 22090277
Article Published Date : Nov 16, 2011
Study Type : Human Study
Diseases : Bisphenol-A Toxicity : CK(46) : AC(10), Insulin Resistance : CK(986) : AC(212), Obesity : CK(1772) : AC(266), Obesity: Abdominal : CK(1611) : AC(56)

National Center for Complimentary & Alternative MedicineHTTP://NCCAM.NIH.GOV/HEALTH/TIPS/YOGA?NAV=FB

Lipoic acid mitigates bisphenol A-induced testicular mitochondrial toxicity in rats.
Click here to see the entire article
Pubmed Data : Toxicol Ind Health. 2012 May 23. Epub 2012 May 23. PMID: 22623521
Article Published Date : May 23, 2012
Study Type : Animal Study
Adverse Pharmacological Actions : Endocrine Disruptor: Testes : CK(1) : AC(1)

Maternal dietary supplementation with methyl donors like folic acid or the phytoestrogen genistein, negated the DNA hypomethylating effect of Bisphenol A - Article 2
Click here to see the entire article
Pubmed Data : Proc Natl Acad Sci U S A. 2007 Aug 7;104(32):13056-61. Epub 2007 : PMID: 17670942
Article Published Date : Aug 07, 2007
Study Type : Animal Study

The brain barrier systems does not limit the access of the lipophilic BPA to the brain.
Pubmed Data : Toxicol Ind Health. 2004 Jun ;20(1-5):41-50. PMID: 15807407
Article Published Date : May 31, 2004
Study Type : Animal Study
Additional Links
Diseases : Bisphenol-A Toxicity : CK(46) : AC(10)
Problem Substances : Bisphenol A : CK(174) : AC(39)
Adverse Pharmacological Actions : Neurotoxic : CK(1064) : AC(179)

The probiotics Bifidobacterium breve and Lactobacillus casei reduce the intestinal absorption of bisphenol A by facillitating its excretion.
Pubmed Data : Biosci Biotechnol Biochem. 2008 Jun;72(6):1409-15. Epub 2008 Jun 7. PMID: 18540113 Pub.Date : Jun 01, 2008
Study Type : Animal Study

Additional Links
Substances : Bifidobacterium : CK(450) : AC(40), Bifidobacterium Breve : CK(57) : AC(9), Lactobacillus casei : CK(151) : AC(26), Probiotics : CK(2370) : AC(235)

Diseases : Bisphenol-A Toxicity : CK(46) : AC(10)
Bisphenol A-glycidyl methacrylate induces a broad spectrum of DNA damage in human lymphocytes.

Pubmed Data : Arch Toxicol. 2011 Nov ;85(11):1453-61. Epub 2010 Sep 29.
PMID: 20878393 Pub Date : Oct 31, 2011
Study Type : In Vitro Study

Weak estrogenic transcriptional activities of Bisphenol A and Bisphenol S.
Pubmed Data : Toxicol In Vitro. 2012 Aug ;26(5):727-31. Epub 2012 Apr 5.
PMID: 22507746 Pub Date : Aug 01, 2012
Study Type : In Vitro Study

A probiotic bacteria found within kimchi known as Bacillus pumilus is capable of degrading bisphenol A.
Pubmed Data : Appl Biochem Biotechnol. 2007 Jan;136(1):39-51. PMID: 17416976   Pub Date : Jan 01, 2007
Study Type : In Vitro Study

Bisphenol A in dental sealants and its estrogen like effect.
Article Publish Status : This is a free article. Pubmed Data : Indian J Endocrinol Metab. 2012 May ;16(3):339-42. PMID: 22629496
Pub Date : May 01, 2012

Bisphenol S has been shown to have estrogenic activity.
Pubmed Data : Toxicol In Vitro. 2001 Aug-Oct;15(4-5):421-5. PMID: 11566573 Pub Date : Aug 01, 2001

Black tea extract and quercetin ameliorate bisphenol A induced cytotoxicity.
Pubmed Data : Acta Pol Pharm. 2009 Jan-Feb;66(1):41-4. PMID: 19226967
Pub Date : Jan 01, 2009

High levels of bisphenol A are found in all world paper currencies tested and are a probably source of exposure.
Pubmed Data : Environ Sci Technol. 2011 Jul 11. Epub 2011 Jul 11. PMID: 21744851 Pub Date : Jul 11, 2011

Royal jelly inhibits the estrogenic and proliferative effect of Bisphenol-A.
Pubmed Data : Biosci Biotechnol Biochem. 2007 Jan;71(1):253-5. Epub 2007 Jan 7. PID:17213647 Pub Date : Jan 01, 2007

A. M. Kaunitz, "Oral Contraceptives," in Thomas G. Stovall and Frank W. Ling, eds., *Gynecology for the Primary Care Physician* (Philadelphia: Current Medicine, 1999).

I. F. Godsland et al., "The Effects of Different Formulations of Oral Contraceptive Agents on Lipid and Carbohydrate Metabolism," New England Journal of Medicine, vol. 323, no. 20 (Nov. 15, 1990), pp. 1375-81.

M. Bernier, Y. Mikaeloff, M. Hudson, and S. Suissa, "Combined Oral Contraceptive Use and the Risk of Systemic Lupus Erythematosus," Arthritis Care & Research, vol. 61, no. 4 (April 15, 2009), pp. 476-81.

V. Cogliano et al., "Carcinogenicity of Combined Oestrogen-Progestagen Contraceptives and Menopausal Treatment," *Lancet Oncology*, vol. 6, no. 8 (August 2005), pp. 552-53.

Collaborative Group on Hormonal Factors in Breast Cancer, "Breast Cancer and Hormonal Contraceptives: Further Results," Contraception, vol. 54, no. 3 suppl. (Sept. 1996), pp. 1S-106S.

Chapter 7

26. Vitamin E For Dysmenorrhoea British Journal of Obstetrics and Gynecology 2001;108:1181-1183
http://www.medicine.ox.ac.uk/bandolier/painres/download/Bando136.pdf

27. Can J Clin Pharmacol. 2009 Fall;16(3):e407-29. Epub 2009 Oct

28. http://www.biomedcentral.com/content/pdf/1472-6882-12-143.pdf

29. Herbs, vitamins and minerals in the treatment of premenstrual syndrome: a systematic review.Whelan AM, Jurgens TM, Naylor H. College of Pharmacy, Dalhousie University, Halifax, Nova Scotia. Anne.Marie.Whelan@Dal.Ca
http://www.ncbi.nlm.nih.gov/pubmed/19923637

30. Am J Obstet Gynecol. 1996 Apr;174(4):1335-8. Supplementation with omega-3 polyunsaturated fatty acids in the management of dysmenorrhea in adolescents. Harel Z, Biro FM, Kottenhahn RK, Rosenthal SL.Division of Adolescent Medicine, Children's Hospital Medical Center, Cincinnati, OH 45229, USA.

31. Getting Enough Calcium in Early Life Could Be Key for Optimal Lifelong Bone Health http://news.ncsu.edu/releases/090dsstahl/

32. http://www.ncbi.nlm.nih.gov/pubmed/20371155

33. Linus Pauling Institute of Micronutrient Research For Optimum Health
    Oregon State University
    http://lpi.oregonstate.edu/infocenter/minerals/zinc/

34 F Facchinetti, P Borella, G Sances, L Fioroni, R E Nappi, A R Genazzani.
    Oral magnesium successfully relieves premenstrual mood changes.
    Obstet Gynecol. 1991 Aug;78(2):177-81. PMID: 2067759

34. A F Walker, M C De Souza, M F Vickers, S Abeyasekera, M L Collins, L A
    Trinca. Magnesium supplementation alleviates premenstrual symptoms
    of fluid retention. *J Womens Health*. 1998 Nov;7(9):1157-65. PMID:
    9861593

34. S Quaranta, M A Buscaglia, M G Meroni, E Colombo, S Cella. Pilot study
    of the efficacy and safety of a modified-release magnesium 250 mg
    tablet (Sincromag) for the treatment of premenstrual syndrome. *Am J
    Gastroenterol*. 2008 Dec;103(12):2972-6. PMID: 17177579

34. M C De Souza, A F Walker, P A Robinson, K Bolland. A synergistic effect
    of a daily supplement for 1 month of 200 mg magnesium plus 50 mg
    vitamin B6 for the relief of anxiety-related premenstrual symptoms: a
    randomized, double-blind, crossover study. *J Womens Health Gend
    Based Med*. 2000 Mar;9(2):131-9. PMID: 10746516

Chapter 8

35. Chinese Herbal Medicine Materia Medica, 3rd Edition, D. Bensky, S.
    Clavey, E. Stoger Eastland Press. 2004

36   Cochrane Database Syst Rev. 2008 Apr 16;(2):CD005288.
Chinese herbal medicine for primary dysmenorrhoea.Zhu X, Proctor M,
    Bensoussan A, Wu E, Smith CA.

Chinese Medicine Program, University of Western Sydney, Center for
    Complementary Medicine Research
    http://www.ncbi.nlm.nih.gov/pubmed/18425916

37 Cochrane Database Syst Rev. 2007 Oct 17;(4):CD005288.
    Chinese Herbal Medicine for Primary DysmenorrhoeaZhu X, Proctor M,
    Bensoussan A, Smith CA, Wu E. Chinese Medicine Program, University of
    Western Sydney, Center for Complementary Medicine Research, Bldg 3,
    Bankstown Campus,Locked Bag 1797, Penrith South DC, Sydney, New
    South Wales, Australia, 2750.x.zhu@uws.edu.au Update in: Cochrane
    Database Syst Rev. 2008;(2):CD005288.

38. J.M. Jellin, F. Batz, K. Hitchens, Pharmacist's Letter/Prescriber's Letter Natural Medicines Comprehensive Database (Stockton, Calif: Therapeutic Research Facility, 1999).

39 Can J Clin Pharmacol. 2009 Fall;16(3):e407-29. Epub 2009 Oct 29.
Herbs, vitamins and minerals in the treatment of premenstrual syndrome: a systematic review.
Whelan AM, Jurgens TM, Naylor H.
http:/www.ncbi.nlm.nih.gov/pubmed/19923637

40 University of Maryland Medical Center
http://www.umm.edu/altmed/articles/menstrual-pain-000052.htm#ixzz254pVgIEh
Chinese herbal medicine for primary dysmenorrhoea.
http://onlinelibrary.wiley.com/doi/10.1002/14651858.CD005288.pub3/abstr act;jsessionid=31CD166DD7556BF3F99B36DAA09162B8.d03t01

41. Clinical Evidence Dysmenorrhoeaearch date January 2010
Pallavi M Latthe, Rita Champaneria, and Khalid S Khan
http://clinicalevidence.bmj.com/x/pdf/clinical-evidence/en-gb/systematic-review/0813.pdf

Clinical efficacy of Kampo medicine (Japanese
traditional herbal medicine) in the treatment of J. Pepping, "Piper methysticum," Am J Health Sys Pharm 56 (1999) : 957-960.

Norra MacReady, "Herb May Curb PMS," Posted 8/7/00 [article online]; available from
http://about.onhealth.com/alternative/news/webmd/item,97089.asp; Internet; cited Sept. 5, 2000.

Tori Hudson, "SOS for PMS," Let's Live, February 2000, 71-74.

Lynn Limon, "Use of Alternative Medicine in Women's Health," Pharmacists Conference Summaries APhA 2000 - American Pharmaceutical Association Annual Meeting, Washington, DC, March 10-14, 2000. [article online]; available from
http://www.medscape.com/medscape/CNO/2000/APHA/APHA-13.html; Internet; cited Sept. 5, 2000.

M. Hardy, "Herbs of special interest to women," J Am Pharm Assoc 40 (2000) : 234-242.

B. Gaster, J. Holroyd, "St John's Wort for depression: a systematic review," Arch Intern Med. 160 (2000) :152-156.

D.F. Horrobin, M.S, Manku, M. Brush, et al., "Abnormalities in plasma essential fatty acid levels in women with premenstrual syndrome and with nonmalignant breast disease," J Nutr Med 2 (1991) : 259–64.

J. Puolakka, L. Makarainen,L. Viinikka, O. Ylikorkola, "Biochemical and clinical effects of treating the premenstrual syndrome with prostaglandin synthesis precursors," J Reprod Med 30 (1985) : 149–53.

P.A. Ockerman, I. Bachrack, S. Glans, S. Rassner, "Evening primrose oil as a treatment of the premenstrual syndrome," Rec Adv Clin Nutr 2 (1986) : 404–405.

H. Massil, P.M.S. O'Brien, M.G. Brush, "A double blind trial of Efamol evening primrose oil in premenstrual syndrome," 2nd International Symposium on PMS, Kiawah Island, Sep 1987.

R. Casper, "A double blind trial of evening primrose oil in premenstrual syndrome," 2nd International Symposium on PMS, Kiawah Island, Sep 1987.

S. K. Khoo, C. Munro, D. Battisutta, "Evening primrose oil and treatment of premenstrual syndrome," Med J Aust 153 (1990) :189–92. A. Collins, A. Cerin, G. Coleman, B. M. Landgren, "Essential fatty acids in the treatment of premenstrual syndrome," Obstet Gynecol 81 (1993) :93–98.

I.J. McFayden, A.P. Forest, et al., "Cyclical breast pain - some observations and the difficulties in treatment," Br J Clin Pract 46 (1992) :161–64.

K. J. Chang, T.T.Y. Lee, G. Linares-Cruz, S. Fournier, and B. de Lingieres, "Influences of Percuntaneous Administration of Estradiol and Progesterone on Human Breast Epithelial Cell Cycle in Vivo," Fertility and Sterility 63 (1995) : 785-791.

John R. Lee, Jesse Hanley and Virginia Hopkins, What Your Doctor May Not Tell You About Premenopause. (New York: Warner Books, 1999), 76-91.

S. L. Plushner, "Valerian: Valeriana officinalis," Am J Health Sys Pharm 57 (2000) :328-335.

V. Ernster, L. Mason, W. Goodson, et. al., "Effects of caffeine-free diet on benign breast disease: A randomized trial" Surgery 91 (1982) 263-267.

Lee et. al, 137-139. Primary dysmenorrhea. Oya A, Oikawa T, Nakai A, Takeshita T, Hanawa T.

Published in : J Obstet Gynaecol Res. 2008 Oct;34(5):898-908.
Department of Obstetrics and Gynecology, Nippon Medical School, Kitasato

Herbal and Dietary Therapies for Primary and Secondary Dysmenorrhoea
Proctor ML, Murphy PA. Department of Obstetrics and Gynaecology, National
Women's Hospital, Claude Road, Epsom, Auckland, New Zealand, 1003.
ml.wilson@auckland.ac.nz

Herbs of Special Interest To Women Hardy ML.J Am Pharm Assoc (Wash).
2000 Mar-Apr;40(2):234-42; quiz 327-9 Cedars-Sinai Integrative Medicine
Medical Group, Cedars-Sinai Hospital, Los Angeles, CA, USA.
HardyM@csmns.org

Chapter 9

Acupuncture for management of primary dysmenorrhea. Obstet Gynecol.
1987 Jan; 69(1):51-6. Helms JM.
Link:http://www.ncbi.nlm.nih.gov/sites/entrez?cmd=search&db=pubmed&te
rm=Helms%20[AU]%20AND%201987%20[DP]%20AND%20Obstet%20Gyn
ecol%20[TA]

Cochrane Database of Systematic Reviews
Source; Zhu X, et al "Chinese herbal medicine for primary dysmenorrhea"
Cochrane Database of Systematic Reviews 2007; 3: CD005288.

Chinese Medicine Program at the University of Western Sydney.1 (fourth
issue for 2007 of The Cochrane Library).

Yin, J. Modern Research and Clinical Application of Chinese Materia Medica
(2) pp 218-219 Beijing:
 R. Hatcher et al., *Contraceptive Technology* (New York: Irvington
Publishers, 1991).

 C. Panzer et al., "Impact of Oral Contraceptives on Sex Hormone Binding
Globulin and Androgen Levels: A Retrospective Study in Women with Sexual
Dysfunction," Journal of Sexual Medicine, vol. 3, no. 1 (January 2006), pp.
104-13.

. M. K. Horwitt et al., "Relationship Between Levels of Blood Lipids, Vitamins
C, A, E, Serum Copper, and Urinary Excretion of Tryptophan Metabolites in
Women Taking Oral Contraceptive Therapy," *American Journal of Clinical
Nutrition*, vol. 28 (1975), pp. 403-12;
K. Amatayakul, "Vitamin Metabolism and the Effects of Multivitamin
Supplementation in Oral Contraceptive Users," Contraception, vol. 30, no. 2
(1984), pp. 179-96; and J. L. Webb, "Nutritional Effects of Oral
Contraceptive Use," *Journal of Reproductive Health*, vol. 25, no. 4 (1980), p.
151.

A case-control study of oral contraceptive use and incident breast cancer.Rosenberg L, Zhang Y, Coogan PF, Strom BL, Palmer JR.Slone Epidemiology Center at Boston University, 1010 Commonwealth Avenue, Boston, MA 02215, USA. lrosenberg@slone.bu.eduAm J Epidemiol. 2009 Sep 15;170(6):802-3; author reply 803-4.

41. Drug-induced liver injury: Is it somehow foreseeable?Giovanni Tarantino, Matteo Nicola Dario Di Minno, Domenico Capone World J Gastroenterol. 2009 June 21; 15(23): 2817–2833. Published online 2009 June 21. doi: 10.3748/wjg.15.2817 PMCID: PMC2698999

The March 2010 issue of the **American Journal of Medicine** contained an analysis of data from 26,000 men, participants in the Health Professionals Follow-up Study. Researchers at Harvard University, Brigham and Women's Hospital, Vanderbilt University, and the Massachusetts Eye and Ear Infirmary, Boston, determined that men younger than 60 who used acetaminophen were 61 percent more likely to experience hearing loss. Studies appearing in the journal **Drug Safety** (2008 Vol 31:pp127-141) have linked acetaminophen to adverse vision events.

American jAssociation of Cancer Research -Long-term use of hormone therapy and breast cancer incidence and mortality Study Apr 01, 2012,

ing lifelong hormonal balance
y every day of the month.

out:

control over your monthly cycle
ance & how to avoid it
's hidden messages
ves to drugs
o the PMS blues

it easy to understand what your
what they are doing. In 10 days or
ll the natural solutions you need to
ur hormones for life. This book is
it women of all ages. Get it today!

olin is a Licensed Acupuncturist, Herbalist and
Oriental Medicine and founder of Pacific Herbs in
California. As a teen she suffered with debilitating
imps and sought out Alternative & Complementary
wers. Through years of personal experience, raising
aughters and treating and counselling patients, she
natives to: "Keep
leash and house
Cathy's motto. Her
dicine perspective
both the root and
ix them forever.

$14.95

ISBN 978-0-9899467-1-1

90000

9 780989 946711

Stop Your BITCHING

CATHY MARGOLIN

Th

End

Build
your body

5.25 x 8.00
203 mm x 133 mm

.420
10.66mm

CPSIA information can be obtained at www.ICGtesting.com
Printed in the USA
LVOW02s1528261013

358745LV00010B/27/P